Unchained and Unbroken

Life Lessons and Strength Training

From a Jailhouse GymRat

Guy W. Gane, Jr.

IngramSpark

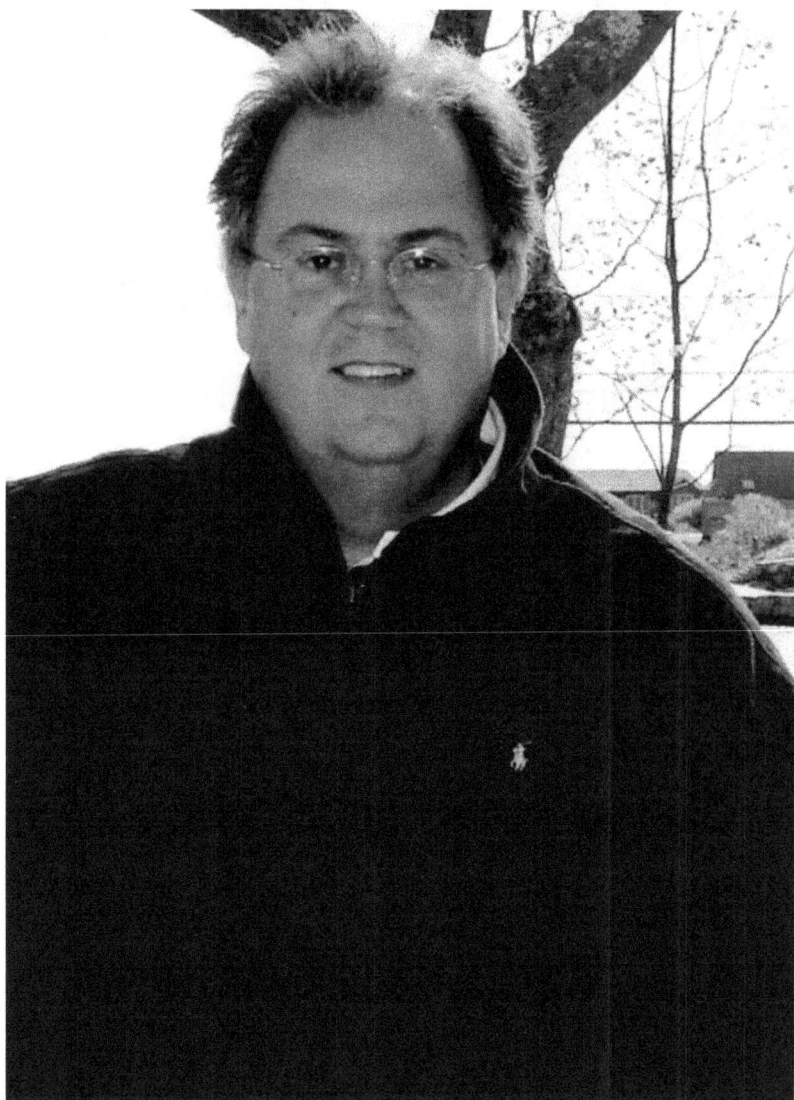

October 2007

"Let's start with a premise that I don't think a lot of Americans are aware of. We have 5% of the world's population; we have 25% of the world's known prison population. We have an incarceration rate in the United States, the world's greatest democracy, that is five times as high as the average incarceration rate of the rest of the world. *There are only two possibilities here: either we have the most evil people on earth living in the United States; or we are doing something dramatically wrong*................"

United States Senator James H. Webb (D, Virginia)

Library of Congress Cataloging-in-Publication Data is available upon request

www.guy@ganewisdom.com

ISBN: 978-0-578-25760-0

This work is non-fiction.

———

Gane, Guy W. Jr

Unchained and Unbroken: Life Lessons and Strength Training from a Jailhouse GymRat

Published: November 2021

2ⁿᵈ Printing: October 2022

To my Children

.

Vi amo tutti oltre le parole

The Glory of God is a Human Being Fully Alive

-St. Irenaeus

INTRODUCTION

He wanted his money. Kicking in the door, the hammer on the Glock cocked and pointed straight at the baby's mother, he yanks the infant from her arms and throws the tiny girl into the microwave. "Give me the money now before I press start."

The mental images are hard to erase and impossible to forget. Hearing the story as he relays it is not only bone chilling but totally sickening.

Another day, another place, another con is at home with his mother and little sister when he hears sounds in another room. Sent by the cartel, the two enforcers are about to carry out the contract when, with feline agility he pumps a shot into each of their foreheads. He left that night, as he relays this story to me, and he's been twenty-seven years in lock-up and thirty years since he last saw his mother. He still has another six to go.

It was common to see guys limping around on the compound, some proud of their narrow escape — and the surgeon's skill — showing me the knife slashes or the bullet's entrance. The OGs, the street guys, and the just plain crazies abound everywhere on the yard.

These men — and many like them — are who I spent nearly nine years in federal prison with. At a time when most guys were planning their retirement, enjoying life with the woman they love, the children they adore, and the grandchildren they treasure, I was forced to plan on how to survive in a subculture of violent tendencies, perceived slights, and rapid mood swings.

The majority of the compound were raised by the streets and have more than a hint of attitude in their voice. Too many of them were doing life on the installment plan and had become institutionalized, losing any semblance of kindness or decency. In order to survive in such an environment, you must earn respect and develop a confident swagger. The best place to acquire both is at the weight pile.

I've tried to spare my readers the gruesome details in the pages that follow. But frankly speaking, in prison there is too much that goes on and goes down, so although you don't have to be an ex con to make a healthy change in your life, that's my perspective, so that's what I'll speak from. Truth be told, I witnessed more than I wished to. Much more. So whether you are a school teacher, a gas station attendant, a customer service representative — or even an ex con — the possibility exists that you can become fit and healthy, even in the midst of personal challenges, regardless of age.

When I entered prison in the fall of 2011, I was a mess — emotionally, mentally, and definitely physically. Weightlifting, cardio training, and core development quite literally saved my life. Experiencing a major health crisis shortly after catching my case in 2008 only exemplified the results of living without regard for my well-being.

I am part of that generation known as the Baby Boomers. We were the ones who ushered in the modern era. We pioneered sit-ins, campus protests, equal rights, disdain for authority, and flower power. We believed (at the time anyway) that "if you're 30, your through!"

We experienced the Beatles, Woodstock, The Cold War, Viet Nam, JFK, and a man walking on the moon. We took so much for granted — not the least of which was our health. Now, ironically, we're the generation that doesn't want to "get old" and have propelled the growth of anti-aging clinics and treatments to assist with that desire.

What I discovered throughout my ordeal is that age is nothing more than a number. I urge you to not focus on your DOB but your YTD — yet to do. If you have been mindful of your health, your diet, and your overall fitness, you are to be applauded. If, however, you were someone like me who neglected his health for years, I have outlined a path to not only wellness but strength and endurance with a formula that can virtually turn back the hands of time.

These methods are not new, but they have been neglected. You see, there was a time in our human story that required us to acquire food from a wild landscape. As hunter-gatherers, our prehistoric ancestors relied on their ability to locate and kill, then carve up and haul back that which they had slain. Meat was how our ancient forbears were able to propagate our species. Although adept at forging nuts, roots and berries, farming as we know it has only been practiced for the last 10,000 years; early man relied on the nutrition provided by what they killed of which protein was a primary nutrient.

What actually allowed humanity to persevere was the physical demands put on the body. Climbing, running, short bursts of speed when

9

necessary, and of course the ability to adapt to the environment, each requiring stamina and ingenuity, characteristics not quite as necessary today as then — prison not withstanding!

Today we rely on organized and specific movements designed to target and develop certain body parts or muscle groups. In a word: exercise.

Exerting the body's musculoskeletal system as well as the central nervous system has many benefits: increased heart health, a heightened immune system, improved brain function, and healthier aging. But what exercises are the best? How long the duration of the workout? To train like a hamster on a wheel going nowhere fast is impressive but quite pointless.

Our diet — what and when — we put into our bodies significantly affects our physical condition, our longevity, and, as research over the last fifty years has discovered, our emotional well-being as well. The good news is that we decide how we fuel our bodies.

We know that energy is expanded by the body's ability to burn calories, known as the metabolic process, which continues every moment. Sitting quietly in a chair consumes eighty calories in an hour's time. That's 1,920 calories every twenty-four hours! Sleeping would expand seventy calories per hour, a moderate-paced walk 200 calories, and an hour of lifting weight at just a manageable pace and effortless weight would burn off 450 calories. These numbers are, of course, affected by your weight, gender, and efficiency of exercise, but it gives you an idea of what your body may be missing out on!

But I didn't know these stats when I started my journey to health. It wasn't about the calories burned. A guy in the joint learns to survive. Emotionally he needs to 'man-up' and the sooner the better. Some guys try to survive by blending into the surroundings, hoping the violent lunatics and psychopaths don't notice them. They eventually do, of course. Some guys look for their homies, thinking guys from the old neighborhood will watch their back. Others become very, shall we say, compliant, in order to do their time and be looked after.

Then there are others who refuse to let the system, circumstances, or another con dominate them. They innovate a no-BS workout-routine, commit to it and get the job done. In this book, you'll find jailhouse-style training routines interspersed with personal observations, anecdotes, and advice gleaned and gathered over the better part of decade of being locked up. Even now I find it incredulous that I spent so many years inside.

Life is full of challenges. Of course, you already know that but meeting those challenges head-on is not the end of it. Instead of avoiding those problems, welcome them. Each test, every trial will strengthen you. They hold nuggets of wisdom that, if you overlook the heartbreak, will cause you to be victorious in the future. Anguish, misery, discomfort, and disappointment are excellent teachers.

The discipline you will learn in the cardio room and in the weight room will extend into every facet of your life if you absorb the lessons and, more importantly, pay attention to them. The workouts, the exercises, the diet, and the habits I developed are found in the pages that follow.

If I could take the broken-down train wreck that I was upon entering federal prison and transform it into a lean, strong, confident, and inspired human being, I am certain that the fundamental principles that

I've enclosed within will do the same for you, no matter the challenges you are facing.

Guy William Gane, Jr.

Chapter 1

"A person often meets his destiny on the road he took to avoid it"

-Jean de La Fontaine

As I walked through the entrance of Federal Correctional Institution (FCI) Elkton, located near Youngstown, Ohio, it was almost as if I could taste the abundance of steel and absorb the vibrations of electricity that surrounded the prison.

"Wake-up! Wake-up! This is only a dream. Open your eyes!" But I was awake. Each beat of my heart reverberated throughout my body, the pressure of the circulation clearly felt. I looked out over an ocean of structures and of barbed wire while at the same time perceiving a sea of anguish inside the sprawling compound. I began to hyperventilate, short bursts of air that barely kept me conscious. Reality however overpowered my comprehension. This *is* prison!

In his masterpiece *The Divine Comedy* Dante Alighieri wrote "Abandon all hope, ye who enter here." And it was those words that began to repeat in my mind as I was led across the prison yard to my unique living quarters.

For some unexplained reason my thoughts kept going back to Dante as I recalled how, when he was banished from his beloved home in Florence and being torn away forever from the woman he adored, he wrote "You shall leave everything you love most."

The same prophesy was now to become mine. How, in God's Mighty name, did this happen?

The odyssey began in 2008.

In July of that year, at the age of fifty-four, I suffered a massive heart attack. Shortly after arriving at the hospital early that July morning I actually checked out. As the ER nurse was fitting an oxygen mask over my face, she said something along the lines of "Welcome back. We lost you. We brought you back with the paddles."

As traumatic as that event was, the more terrifying ordeal I was experiencing at that moment was being pursued by the US Government — the guys that won World War II.

As a stockbroker for many years, I witnessed the dramatic rise of the Dow Jones from 577 in 1974 to over 11,500 by 2006. It was in that year that I, along with two investment bankers recalibrated the brokerage firm I personally owned into a company that we named WaterMark. Raising capital for operating expenses for the new company eventually brought the firm, and I, to the attention of the Securities and Exchange Commission and to the US Attorney's office as well.

Ultimately after several years of trying to convince the prosecutors of my innocence to the charges of money-laundering and mail fraud, I stood before a federal judge who handed me a bone-crushing sentence of thirteen years on the two counts. I spent what in the end became eight years, nine months and five days in prison. I decided early in my sentence that I would focus on the only things I could still control in my life: my body and my mind. With an iron-willed determination, I set out to do exactly that. As I dejectedly made my way across the compound, I knew I would need to transform my fifty-seven-year-old body into a physical structure that could withstand the years ahead.

Every generation, it seems, wants to discover how to develop and maintain not only health and vitality but strength and youth as they age. Forced to uncover this mystery, I learned the method to do so. I developed a formula for enjoying the years ahead, full of life and limitless enthusiasm, despite the challenges I would come to face. This method for not only getting healthy, but for recalibrating your mind — no matter your age — to tackle any obstacles in front of you.

It is said that your reality is what you perceive it to be and your attitude towards an event determines your reaction towards it. Prison is no joke. It is not possible to say "I don't like it here. I'm leaving!" If there is a hell on earth, prison comes near to it. You are forced to live with every manner of personality—murderers, cartel leaders, drug dealers, violent gang members, rapists, pimps, child pornographers and molesters, as well as psychopaths and psychotics. Every new arrival is scrutinized by these rogues and impressions are quickly being formed.

Early on, other inmates conclude if you are the predator or if you are the prey. You're sized up and judged as someone who can be messed with or someone who should be left alone. Your walk, your posture, your physique, your total body language all broadcast if you are easy pickings or not. As a new arrival you better be prepared to be tested, if not hassled, soon after entering GP - general population. Prison is full of Alpha Males, guys who are used to doing things their way and above all demand to be shown deference to.

Respect is a big deal behind bars. Although inwardly you may not feel that toward another con you sure as hell better not show that you don't. What seems trivial on the street, on the outside — like picking up a magazine on an otherwise empty chair — can get you hurt. Accidently bumping into someone better be quickly followed by a sincere apology else a rock-hard fist slams into the back of your head like a sledgehammer.

You must constantly be aware of what is going on and going down around you. Your reaction to what's happening is also noted by the more belligerent in the group. The guys in the yard will notice if you're "all show or no go" at once. They'll look to see if you're "battle-ready." Big biceps alone — the showy stuff the pretty boys work on at the designer gym — won't cut it. A guy's back, his shoulders, his quads, his calves, his neck, his forearms — these are what a con checks out when he decides to assault you or avoid you. While I obviously didn't have any experience in a women's prison, I imagine the same is true.

When I walked through those massive prison gates all those years ago, I was a very soft 248 pounds. Prior to the heart attack I clocked in at a hefty 286 pounds! Although I had been a power lifter for years, I allowed my career to overtake the time I worked out, and by 2003 when I chose to take a lay-off from lifting, I began to work even longer hours, become ever more stressed and eat terribly. In short, I was in sorry shape.

What followed was a choice to bring my body back into health. My path to wellness and strength brought an abundance of tears. Tears of frustration, tears of desperation, and tears of loss. But along with the grief, I gained wisdom and a strength of character that I never knew I possessed. I gained a broad perspective of life that, quite truthfully, I would have rather not experienced. In the same breath however, I am eternally grateful for the trial.

My motivation to begin strength training again was to be in a position to defend myself. I was older than most of the other inmates (forty-one years old being the average age) which could cause me to be considered a pushover. I knew that could not fly. My driving force to get healthy, in addition to holding my own against an aggressor, was to have the strength and stamina needed to work toward repaying those who lost money with my company. The saddest outcome of being incarcerated was that those investors were in jail with me, knowing that as long as I was locked up, they had no-one committed to repay them.

Being overweight and out of shape for so long, my first thought after entering prison was "I need to lose weight." I also suffered with chronic back pain. When I was on the outside, I was able to get to the chiropractor when the need arose, which was a few times a month. Back pain can be caused by and exacerbated by a weak core. So not only was my abdomen weak and out of shape, but I was squatting heavy back then, my PR – personal record – being 500 pounds. Putting excess weight, which in this case was bearing down on my spine, on an already stressed back was not wise. Before I could begin to lift again, I needed to start foundationally. Losing weight became goal number one.

Behind the fence there are a lot of guys moving huge weights. You look at a guy with an enormous neck and thick traps, shoulders the size of coconuts and legs like Corinthian pillars and you know he means business. He's big, he's brawny, he's strong as hell. But inside, his cardiovascular system could be a mess. I saw guys who were able to walk into the weight pit and pull a 455-pound deadlift with ease. It was their bulk that assisted in the lift. In plain English, they were big but they lacked endurance. I also saw guys that were the real deal - strong and fit. They knew, as I did, that to be truly in shape they needed to do everything right. That starts in the cardio room.

Moving iron correctly is work. It is the result of good conditioning. For a person who wants to develop a strong core, lift heavy, be healthy, achieve genuine endurance, and look good they need to include cardio work. To a lot of cons being strong is all that matters, however what good is all that muscle if it's hidden by layers of fat? More importantly though, if their cardiovascular system is a mess, how athletic or healthy are they really?

Cardio work is difficult. It takes time — lots of it — to begin to see results. It takes dedication —an hour or more three times a week at the least. It hurts. You must learn to tune out the little devil on your shoulder telling you "You can do this tomorrow" or "Just do another minute" when you have another ten to go. "Why bother?" You get the picture.

The simplest cardio work you can perform is walking. I observed a great number of guys in lock-up who hit the track and trudged two, three, four, even as many as twelve miles a day. Marching around the track afforded you some 'alone time' but it also took off weight. Guys dropped twenty or thirty pounds over a period of a few months. One of my buddies, Jason, walked six miles a day taking him about two and a half hours. He lost over thirty pounds within four months.

Most inmates who were seriously into weightlifting would be found in the cardio room. Personally, I was in the cardio room five times a week, eventually ratcheting up to six days a week. It became an unexpected habit that I came to enjoy. There were weeks when I needed to rein myself in for fear of overtraining, as I would be eager to work out there every day as well as at the weight pit. I knew of guys who did workout everyday — some twice a day. In a short time, those inmates stopped growing. We'll talk about overtraining later.

On the outside, in the free world, you have the option of choosing what machines to buy, what gym to workout at, what time you go there, how long you stay. Behind the fence a con's time is very structured and you use whatever equipment is available — if it's not broken. Despite these possible hitches a lot of impressive physiques walk out of the joint. It comes down to commitment not commiseration.

My work schedule allowed me to get my cardio workout done in the morning generally lasting from 7:30 until 9 or 9:30 a.m. Afternoons at 1:30 found me at the weight pile and usually lasted an hour.

Since there were plenty of guys trying to grab the same few cardio machines, my workouts were focused, intense, and efficient. Three ellipticals, two treadmills, a stationary bike, a rowing machine, a slant (sit-up) rack, and a Roman bench made up the contents of the room. A pull-up bar and yoga mats were also available. Although the equipment was generally quite old, it did the job if it was working.

The How and Why of the Cardio Room

At a gym, you're able to climb on a state-of-the-art machine, a treadmill let's say, and begin a program tailored to your needs. Most health clubs have calculations available to design a workout that will allow weight and fat loss. In prison, you get on and work your tail off, judging by a look at the scale every day to see if things are coming together for you. When I first stepped on an elliptical, I struggled to stay on for five minutes! But having made the personal commitment to lose weight, I stuck with it. After a week (working out three times a week when I first entered prison in 2011) I was up to eight minutes. Soon it was fifteen minutes, and after a few months, an hour and more. Within twelve months my weight went from 248 pounds to 187! A loss of sixty-one pounds.

Although weights weren't available at Elkton, I stayed focused on my training and felt that were I to be transferred to another prison eventually that did have weights, I would be prepared. Unfortunately, an increasing number of the nation's prisons are removing weights from their compound. Since you're on the outside, you may have preconceived ideas (as I did before the nightmare began) that guys behind bars pack on pounds of muscle, get totally (and outrageously) ripped, get out of prison, and prey on the weak. Can I say this doesn't happen? No. But it is nowhere near what the public believes.

There are a lot of frustrated, unhappy, and lonely convicts in jail. The ability to lift, to train their bodies, takes what otherwise would be negative pent-up energy and release that into a positive endeavor that builds a foundation of discipline and does nothing but improve a guy's character and attitude.

As the years went by, I was finally transferred to another prison facility (via Con-Air) and fortunately there were weights there. Once there, I continued to train in the cardio room but I eventually discovered a vastly superior method of performing cardio work — what's known as HIIT (High Intensity Interval Training).

When we exercise, we would like to know that we're doing something for a purpose, knowing that there are tangible benefits. Sure, we'll receive positive comments from others but when we examine the physiological effects that cardio training has on our bodies, we can appreciate the exceptional results from doing so.

As we age, tiny particles in the cells of our bodies, known as ribosomes, begin to diminish. These particles contribute to protein synthesis (combining elements into a whole) and muscle building. Many conditions which are categorized as "age-related" diseases begin at the cellular level. In order to examine the advantages that exercise has on the cellular level we should be aware of how we benefit from the exercise and then apply that knowledge effectively.

The body is constructed in such a way that it can usually withstand occasional minor illnesses, injuries, and disturbances — inconsequential falls, bumps, and bruises come to mind. However, exceptional health and significant strength can only be built on a solid foundation. Our cell's mitochondrial capacity (which is the amount of fuel accessible to nourish mitochondria) responds well to intense exercise. Mitochondria are the source of energy in the cell and focusing on this particular specialized cell-part can produce tremendous age-related results. One of the means to accomplish this is through HIIT.

For many years, it was thought that doing intensive cardio work ate up muscle and many of the guys training on the sands in California had a real fear toward cardio for this reason. Track athletes, specifically sprinters, developed solid musculature while reducing fat through a combination of calorie-burning workouts. The weight training and the powerlifting communities began to take notice.

HIIT combines short blasts of extreme effort with periods of lighter activity, HIIT is the only type of cardio training that promotes lean muscle growth while releasing growth hormones and increasing the body's metabolic rate. In addition, research has shown that the metabolic burn from HIIT can go on for up to seventeen hours, as compared to three to six hours with a lighter cardio workout! This kind of training has also been found to assist athletes to lighten their total intake of oxygen. All this with as little as twenty to thirty minutes of power exercise!

Behind the fence, anytime you are able to grab a spot in the cardio room it's considered fortunate. With hundreds, even thousands of guys anxious to get in their time as well, it is a good idea to get there, get your work in, and get out. Too many street guys have no problem making your workout (and your life) miserable. Unless you can back up your reprimand for being a jerk or for running their mouth, you keep quiet. My feeling is that if your singing, talking, or rapping you're not working out. When you've got enough breath to babble, you're wasting energy. By the time I left prison I had enough "cred" with everyone that the big mouths were usually respectful and kept quiet. Working out was my escape from prison and the simple fact was that I didn't want to be bugged.

HIIT sessions lend themselves to time limits perfectly. If I wanted respect, I also had to show it, especially when it came to time.

What's great about HIIT is that the sessions are blasted out, usually in fifteen minutes on a specific exercise. You get on, go all out and move on to the next machine. What really makes this kind of training even more effective is the tremendous effect it has on our DNA. Specifically, on what are known as telomeres.

Telomeres are the protein caps that protect chromosomes. Telomeres shrink as we age and each time a cell divides, we lose bits of them. These biological markers are like the plastic tips you'd find on a shoelace. Those people with shorter telomeres, according to research done over the last several years, are found to die sooner. These people are more prone to develop many of the chronic diseases that are commonly found in society. Research has also found that those who exercise strenuously — think thirty- to forty-minute HIIT sessions four to five days per week — have longer telomeres. This research also put forth the idea that strenuous exercise could preserve these protein caps by reducing the stress and inflammation from our daily lives.

I hope you'll forgive me for this dry explanation on the value of HIIT but, as these studies suggest, vigorous exercise can actually slow the aging process on a cellular level and has the capability to literally turn back the hands of time *BY NEARLY A DECADE*, according to this research! If you've been doing HIIT cardio training, great! Likely, however, you picked up this book to learn about how to begin or excel your journey to health, so let's talk about how to get started.

First, plan on the long game. By that I mean be realistic. Although research has shown that HIIT, resistance training, or a mix of light weight training and steady cycling over a twelve-week period help sedentary adults become more fit, HIIT has been shown to be much more beneficial. When you step on an elliptical for the first time, for instance, try to work up to five minutes. Do this three times a week for two weeks. After six workouts, you'll know whether eight minutes is doable. Work up to ten minutes three times a week and fifteen minutes within six weeks. Consistency is important. Continue until you reach thirty minutes. You may advance faster or slower than these suggestions. You are pacing yourself. Before too long you will discover your conditioning level improving. This schedule is also suitable to the treadmill, rowing machine, or stationary bike.

By the tenth week, if not before, you will have worked up your cardio endurance sufficiently to begin HIIT. Again, I remind you, be realistic. Allow your body time to develop into this training, schedule and commitment. Keep in mind: This is for you!

What you are looking for with HIIT is a steady pace for forty-five seconds and a maximum effort for fifteen seconds. Some trainers will have their students work with different time intervals. I use the traditional method of HIIT, hence this pace. If you are using a bicycle for HIIT, use only a stationary bike! When I shared this program with one of my closest friends, Alex, who was among the land of the free, he chose to ride his bike on pavement while performing HIIT. During the workout he hit something, not knowing what, and went airborne, almost killing himself. He sent me pictures of his totally destroyed bike and beaten-up body. It was awful. A stationary bike will allow you to focus on your workout rather than your surroundings.

When performing HIIT, pay strict attention to the seconds. Keep your environment disturbance-free during this time! If your goal is weight-loss, perform HIIT at least four days per week for at least fifteen minutes. If the objective is weight maintenance, three days should be sufficient. Along with proper nutrition, which we'll address shortly, these plans work.

If you've thought about running (not to be confused with escaping!) in the past but felt challenged as to how to start without losing enthusiasm eventually, here is a method I used with success. You will need a stopwatch. Run for thirty seconds, walk for three minutes. Give yourself two weeks and three times per week, with rest days every other day. During the third week, run for sixty seconds, walk for three minutes. During the fifth week, run for ninety seconds, walk for ninety seconds. During the sixth week, run for two minutes, walk for one minute. By the eighth week, set a goal and run without a break. By this point, one mile should be very doable. You may be able to advance more quickly than this schedule, or you may need to take things more slowly. Like every type of exercise, you will be competing against yourself, and consistency is the important factor in achieving any goal.

If you have access to a rowing machine, you have one of the most complete exercise apparatuses available. A rower allows you to engage the back, legs, shoulders, and arms as well as an intense cardio workout if you wish. The goal on this machine is a steady pace for the first seven to ten days, giving your body the opportunity to adjust to the workout. After that, perform an all-out power stroke for thirty seconds with one minute recovery — meaning you slow your pace, not stop the movement. Unless you are an experienced rower, it's advisable to stay at level one (most machines go to ten) for a HIIT cardio workout. Look to accomplish eight minutes with this routine to start off.

Using the HIIT method, the goal is a fifteen-minute workout, with forty-five seconds steady pace and fifteen-seconds of maximum effort. Within a few months you might want to consider a circuit training with one or more of the above exercises. Consider: Fifteen minutes on the rowing machine and fifteen minutes on the elliptical, for instance. Unless your goal is to drop a considerable amount of weight within a relatively short amount of time, a fifteen-minute HIIT session on any one machine is sufficient. If you opt to run, you will want to sprint for short burst of fifteen seconds and walk for forty-five seconds. Regardless of how you break up your high intensity interval training, you will quickly develop enhanced stamina and endurance. Again: Be consistent. Constantly challenge yourself. This is for you, no one else.

Chapter 2

The best medicine for the heart is sweat……

Personally, the euphoria of being in the zone in my training — both cardio and weight — overcame any pain or discomfort I may have had. It was my escape from prison, as I said. I became absorbed in the exercise I was performing, and not only did I feel a sense of accomplishment but also of gratification that I was making positive changes to my body. In prison, time can be overwhelming. Not only was I away from those I loved, but I was forced to live with people I would not normally associate with. Anything that took me out of that place mentally was a good thing. It was an added bonus that working out sent a message to the carnivores on the compound.

There is an exhilaration you find from leaving "nothing on the table" and that was an objective that I embraced. Although the weight pit was the center of life for the guys who worked out, the cardio room was where the lean, toned bodies were fashioned. As we discussed in the last chapter, cardio builds the solid foundation where a granite-like physique can become possible. For the truly committed, the person who has gained proficiency and mastery of training hard and training intensely, there is another level of discipline (and that's what training is) that brings an enormous degree of indefatigability, toughness, and strength: The Tabata Method.

In 1996 Izumi Tabata, an assistant coach of the Japanese Olympic Speed Skaters, found that eight twenty-second rounds of intense work, followed in turn by ten seconds of rest, had the capability to greatly improve anaerobic (the absence of free oxygen) capacity and VO_2 Max (maximal oxygen intake or the measurement of the maximum amount of oxygen a person can use during intense exercise).

In 2013 the American Council on Exercise decided to conduct its own independent research of this four-minute technique. This study, done in conjunction with the University of Wisconsin, La Crosse, found that during a Tabata-style workout, subjects averaged 86 percent of their maximum heart rate and 74 percent of their maximum VO_2. The researchers found that Tabata HIIT met or exceeded established industry guidelines for improving cardiovascular fitness and modifying body composition. Because this is a very intense workout, it should only be used by those with a fairly high level of fitness and no more than two to three times per week, forty-eight to seventy-two hours apart.

Behind the razor wire there is an atmosphere of danger that's always present. At any given moment trouble can erupt. As an inmate, you try to avoid problems, but unfortunately problems generally find you. In lock-up you are forced to be on guard. You learn to keep one eye open when you're sleeping. Prison is comparable to a jungle but instead of the sound of cracking twigs you detect the sound of feet. You acquire an awareness of sounds out of the ordinary. You obtain an extra sense, a mental agility almost above and beyond what's needed in the free world. And most importantly you come to the party prepared. I trained for such parties.

When you train, train hard. Train with purpose and intensity. Be serious about your workout. Although you will never see the inside of a jail cell (my wish for you) and need to defend yourself from a belligerent desperado, you may come into contact with a jackass with an attitude or a bigmouth without a filter. It would be sensible to possess the strength and stamina to be prepared. This is why most cons get jacked up. It's the law of the jungle.

Be disciplined. If you've been inattentive to your body, your health, your strength, or your life, begin now to reverse the neglect. You can do this! Each of us are unique. Your body will respond, as well as perform, differently than the next person. Your fitness level is distinct and dissimilar to others, so I encourage you to keep your workout goals and objectives to yourself. The only person you should compete against is you.

Keep a journal of every workout, cardio or weightlifting. Years ago, when I began lifting, my trainer (and cherished friend) John Carnduff, advised me to write every workout down—the exercise performed, the number of sets, and reps as well as any nuances. For instance, "right shoulder cramped on eighth rep of fourth set of military press" or " left knee — patella — hurting on leg press" or " EZ Curl bar preacher: 125 pounds. Eight times. Personal Record!" Any notes allow you to measure challenges and successes as well as your sticking points. The great advantage of keeping a journal of your workouts is viewing your progress.

Bring your journal with you to the gym and don't feel strange if you are the only person that has done so. I was teased constantly by the other cons because I wrote everything down. I never paid them no mind. Actually, I have all of the journals I kept in prison since the day I began training again. John has been gone many years now but what he taught me so long ago still holds true today "You'll never know how far you can go without a map to help get you there." The journal is your map.

Working out at a fitness center or gym on the outside is less intimidating than in lock-up. In a prison yard there is an abundance of testosterone at the weight pile. Every con knows that when they set foot in a workout area for the first time they will be kept under surveillance. Your physique, your form, your technique, everything will be observed. They also know that you only get to make a first impression once. Ego, pridefulness, respect, all of this play a role in a first-time appearance. How you handle this "audition" will determine your even being allowed in the space again. It's not uncommon to see guys chased-out of a weight or cardio room, and once you're thrown out you stay out. Or else.

But on the outside, you have just as much a right to be in the gym as anyone else there. Though it may feel intimidating for first timers, you will be physically safe, and there is likely to be gym staff to assist you if you have questions about a machine.

As human beings we tend to believe that our heart is the center of our personal existence. We also instinctively believe that our emotions are anchored there, hence phrases such as "he wears his heart on his sleeve," " he's a big-hearted guy," " the heart of the problem" and so on. Although the phrase "cardio work" is spoken about often, some folks know little as to how to build that part of our anatomy into a powerful structure able to deliver staying power and toughness to the rest of the body. A bit larger than the size of your fist, your heart is a muscular organ that needs to be worked properly and the most effective way to accomplish this is through exercise.

Behind the wall I saw guys who were strong as hell quickly fall back in a fight due to a lack of aerobic endurance. They became winded quickly. Actually, the street guy who knew how to tune somebody up would usually fall back and let their opponent use up their energy and endurance by swinging wildly, exhausting themselves quickly.

A prison fight is not a couple of guys trading a few slaps or even a few punches. There are no Marquee of Queensbury rules; in fact, there are no rules at all. This is not a dust-up but a very real duel that can (and sometimes does) end badly. The real American Gladiators are not on some Hollywood sound stage, they are housed in America's prisons.

I realized that I had to be ready to take care of myself, and when I walked through those steel prison gates in the fall of 2011, I was far from being ready. Once I witnessed what goes on behind razor wire, cold stone walls, and locked three-inch-thick iron doors, I knew what I had to do.

I had a bit of "lead time" in that I had a group of guardian angels watching my back at Elkton. The 'made guys'— those you know as organized crime figures — kept an eye out for me. Being Italian (my true family name is Iovannisci) was always something I have taken great pride in, but suddenly it was what was keeping me safe. Once I was transferred out of FCI Elkton a few years later, however, I was on my own.

Although I found my way to the cardio room at Elkton, it was more to lose weight than to build bulk. It wasn't until I was transferred to Northeast Pennsylvania to FCI Schuylkill that I truly understood how dangerous prison really is. There, it was necessary not only bulk up but to strengthen my core, become extremely agile, and work at an intensity level I could not have imagined on the outside. And at fifty-nine years old (at the time of my transfer) I not only wished I could turn back the hands of time, I proceeded to do exactly that. High intensity workouts which included the Tabata Method, crunches, push-ups, yoga and now, thankfully, weights, became my focus. Out of my survival instinct, working out actually came to define me.

You don't need to be in prison to want to drastically change your life, but my time allowed me the mental awakening to do just that. In Chapter 4, we'll talk about the methods I developed to quickly get jacked up in a minimal amount of time. Instead of high-tech machines, you'll be able to use your body weight and pig-iron to get massively strong and possess the capacity to endure beyond your previous expectations.

The bullies you encounter in life are best to be avoided. But when retreat is not an option, you will be prepared. Weather it's the loudmouth at the grocery checkout, the chump checking out your girl, or the jackass who plays the office tough guy, you'll be equipped to do the job.

But before we can get jacked, your body needs the right fuel.

Nutrition

There are hundreds of books on the market concerning nutrition. But I've got a different perspective — the perspective of an ex-con. In the joint you make do. With a lot. You make do with rules and regulations. You make do with the other inmates. You make do with seeing those you love only once in a while. You make do with the food you're served.

There are two topics that are near and dear to most every inmate's heart. Food is the second. Guys talk about food, dream about it, obsess about it and think about it. Constantly. They talk about the dishes they miss, the tastes they remember, but what they miss the most is sharing meals with those they love. They talk about " back when" and "when I get out..." After a few years I found myself cutting out recipes! I would envision the day I could eat something that actually tasted good and was enjoyable to eat.

You've likely taken much of what you eat, the company you keep at dinner time and the chance to enjoy a night out highlighted by a candle-lit dinner, for granted. Don't. Be mindful of the experience. Above all be thankful for every moment. As I sadly discovered those experiences don't last forever.

The human body is nothing if not a bundle of miraculous intricacies all working divinely together to sustain its own viability. The body incorporates three energy-producing systems to create power or, in other words, energy. This first source is known as the ATP/PC cycle — a cellular respiration process that converts food energy. Primarily associated with anaerobic exercise, this energy system lasts from zero to sixty seconds. Secondly, the lactic acid — a syrupy acid found in blood and muscle tissue — cycle system burns mostly sugar and can last from forty-five seconds to five minutes. The third system, known as the Beta-oxidative — a process by which fatty acid molecules are broken down — cycle can last from four minutes to infinity.

With all these systems in mind, it's important to note that eating prior to a cardio workout is actually counterproductive. A meal consisting of carbs or sugars will cause the body to burn them as energy sources *before* it burns fat stores held there. The body finds it easier to burn carbohydrates as opposed to burning fats due to the heat and oxygen required to burn those fats. This is a reason that it takes several minutes before the fat burning process starts when you begin your workout. Science has confirmed that lunchtime is the point of the day that the body requires the largest amount of energy necessary to keep the temperature of the body up. In other words when you eat lunch less energy proceeds into fat - reserves!

There are many supplements on the market that claim to expedite the process of burning fat. We will discuss supplements in the next chapter, but for now, understand that rather than spend money needlessly on such products, you could wear layered clothing when you work out which would heighten fat burning abilities.

In prison it seems you are never given enough to eat. In fact, one of the kitchen guards at Elkton was quoted as saying (and meaning), "If I had my way you guys would get bread and water." I imagine a fair percentage of American citizens might share the same opinion. However, the fact is inmates are generally served small-portioned, high-starch, carbohydrate-loaded meals with white rice being one of the most common provisions. It's probably served at least half-a-dozen times per week. Sometimes more. As starchy foods metabolize to sugar, diabetes, obesity and high blood pressure are endemic to those behind bars. Conversely however there is a positive aspect to prison meals due to the strict time schedule for breakfast, lunch, and dinner. It is a bit easier for an inmate to plan a workout around those pre-set times as well as counting on a certain amount of carbs, proteins, and fats derived those meals.

There are a multitude of companies that offer weight-loss assistance. Many, if not most, cost hundreds or thousands of dollars. The challenge, however, is keeping the weight off after you've left the program. It will take discipline to be successful in both losing weight and maintaining the weight loss. Anything worthwhile takes commitment and consistency. It is not only possible to lose weight, but also definite if you are committed and consistent.

Guys behind bars don't have anything to work with except willpower. They, like you, make a choice. But, of course, unlike you they face a live-or-die decision if they choose to do nothing. You, while hopefully not in a life-or-death situation, have far more temptations and ease of access to unhealthy nutrition options. As such, you will need discipline.

In prison, you eat what you're served, but the ideal diet would include high-quality, low-calorie foods. Each of us need those foods to be full of the necessary vitamins and minerals. Unfortunately, the average food intake of a person in the developed world far exceeds what our bodies need or can burn off on a daily basis. The advantage you have living in freedom is the ability to tailor your diet, what foods to eat, and how to prepare that food. Cons can only control their diet by buying the few nutritious choices at the commissary, skipping meals (even taking into account the modest portions given at mealtime), or by fasting— either a total fast or intermittent fasting. We'll discuss this more later.

Unlike an inmate, you have control over your diet, which means you can ensure you are getting the proper nutrients for your body's essential functions. As an example, let's talk about insulin. Insulin is essential for the normal function of our brain. However, as we age, our bodies have the tendency to become insulin resistant. (In addition to aging, our diets also promote insulin resistance, especially in the United States.) Staples in the American diet like refined carbohydrates and beef, for instance, contribute to this resistance. Lack of exercise and obesity also increase the likelihood of insulin resistance.

Beef is rarely fed to guys on the inside therefore the instances of insulin resistance is somewhat minimized, but not by much due to the other foods served. Chicken in some form is the food of choice by most prison facilities. Although carbs are served in abundance, they can be consciously avoided if an inmate so chooses.

Inactivity is generally not an option in the American Penal System. Of course, there are guys who do nothing but eat and lay around, but the compounds are expansive, and it is not unusual to walk long distances in order to get to your assigned destination before the doors are locked. For the inmate who lacks motivation to exercise, and there are quite a few, there are still stairs to climb, long distances to walk, and work assignments to complete.

On the outside, it is much easier to be sedentary, depending on your lifestyle and job. That is how I got into such poor shape to begin with. I gave up weight training and put in many more hours at my sedentary job. So the discipline you began to learn in your cardio exercises from the first chapter will continue to prove helpful as you begin to change your eating habits in the future.

There are biochemical mechanisms built into each of us that help us acquire and store food so that during lean times this stored energy can be used for repairing our body and resisting stress on it. When we fast, mechanisms are released which promote built-in cell-renewal. Generally, calorie restriction, but more specifically carbohydrate restriction, assists our body to overcome insulin resistance which forces our brain to forgo glucose (which, as you'll remember, is an energy source the brain needs) and become dependent on ketone, a back-up fuel. There is a complicated transformation that takes place in the body in order for these exchanges to happen, but simply put, the brain is protected during periods of starvation.

Unintentionally, our twenty-first century diets have brought about many of the chronic diseases prevalent in today's world. Fortunately, we can reverse much of this harm through periodic intermittent fasting. Cellular reprogramming, revitalized glucose metabolism, and a general feeling of wellness can be accomplished by retraining yourself to eat at specific times and limiting those times when you do.

I have used total fasting and intermittent fasting to achieve specific health goals. To be candid, fasting is less complicated in prison than on the street. There is no significant other on the yard that must adjust their life, diet, or eating habits to accommodate yours. The family is not disrupted by being forced to eat at a specified time in order for you to meet your goal. And the most important point that we touched on earlier: There are many temptations at home. When I finally came home, I was truly overwhelmed by the food available. (The technology too, but that's another story!). I had forgotten, it seemed, what great-tasting food was like. What is similar between being locked up or free, however, is the willpower. How badly do you want to achieve your objective? That said, let's go through a variety of diets that can help you achieve your health goals.

The 16:8 Diet

The 16:8 diet is one that will take a bit of adjustment to your eating schedule. It will also take a moderate amount of willpower but it certainly is doable. During an eight-hour period you will eat as you normally do. Other than pigging out, you can eat what and how much (to satisfy your hunger) you want. The remaining sixteen hours you can drink water, black coffee, and tea. Nothing more than this. If this seems like work, it is. But keep this in mind: You are also asleep for about half of that time. If you forgo breakfast and wait for lunch you will have expanded the full sixteen hours, provided you stop eating after 7 p.m. You will see results within a few weeks doing this program three to four times a week. I continue to use this diet to maintain my weight.

In 2012 the Salk Institute in California reported in the journal "Cell Metabolism" the research they conducted covering sixteen-hour fasting.

A group of mice were fed a high-fat diet around the clock for 18 weeks. This resulted in these mice developing fatty livers, pancreatic disease and diabetes.

Another group of mice were fed *THE EXACT SAME NUMBER OF CALORIES PER DAY* but in an 8 hour window only. The second group *STAYED SLIMMER AND IN BETTER HEALTH FOR A MUCH LONGER PERIOD OF TIME!*

The 5:2 Diet

If limiting your food consumption into a set time seems too restrictive, another plan known as the 5:2 diet might be worth exploring.

This plan, plain and simple, will take real willpower and commitment. This option requires a person to eat normally for five days and to limit themselves to 600 calories a day for the other two. Here you must make smart food choices. Remember, if you cheat you are only cheating yourself. On these two days it would be wise to eat protein-packed small meals including those foods shown to be low calorie but highly satiating.

This diet is designed to drop weight quickly and boasts of being the diet of choice for those in the entertainment business. The two days do not need to be consecutive. You could break them up during the week, but to be effective it is important to establish a schedule and stick to that schedule.

The FMD Diet

Known as the **Fasting Mimicking Diet**, this plan is designed to trick the body by lowering calorie intake to 1,100 calories on the first day and lowering calorie consumption to 800 per day the next four. This need only be done once a month.

Total Fast

The word autophagy is from the Greek meaning "self-devouring." When we eat, our body releases insulin. This release disrupts the process of autophagy which essentially deconstructs old, damaged ingredients in order to release energy and create new molecules.

Autophagy intercedes to offset the aging of cells and assists in building immunity. *Fasts provoke autophagy* according to research done at the University of Graz in Austria in 2017.

This plan is an all-out fast. While there is strong evidence that total fasting has enormous benefits. along with receiving those advantages comes discomfort. This diet is only for those serious about shedding pounds and genuinely committed to improving their health.

Known as therapeutic fasting, this program calls for performing a five-day fast, one to three times a year, and *could* purge any pre-cancerous cancer cells that may be drifting in your body. Done in conjunction with deep prayer and meditation will bring you into a very spiritual and illuminating experience. [2]

It is essential that you stay well hydrated during any type of fast and *critical* during a total fast. A daily multivitamin should also be included. This fast would be best spread out during the year in conjunction with fasts of forty-eight to seventy-two hours monthly.

With any of these fasts you likely will experience a feeling of slight dizziness. This is especially noticeable if you're lying down and quickly jump to your feet. Incorporating intermittent fasting with cardio training not only will enhance cardiovascular health but will aid in effective weight loss.

Cardio training is most effective when selective oxidation (where fatty acid molecules are broken down) of body fat is at the greatest. Knowing when that is, knowing what foods to eat, knowing what foods to limit or avoid, and knowing the optimal time to do all of this is consequential.

If you eat carbohydrates before (and/or/during) cardio training the fuel source being used are from the carbohydrates rather than the fats as we discussed earlier. In a fasted state, performing cardiovascular exercise (as well as weightlifting, if done at a fast pace) maximizes body fat loss. Simply put, exercise that is done in a fasted state causes molecular changes in the muscle cells that causes fat to be used as fuel. Glycogen, the principal storage carbohydrate, is the body's first choice of its source of energy. Fasting seriously diminishes this source.

Not having access to the internet when I was locked up prevented me from investigating into high-protein, low-fat recipes. Although I would not have had these foods available anyway, it would have given me an idea of what those foods were. Instead, I became near obsessive to find other more traditional venues from which to learn them. Some of the more cerebral of the inmates would leave science journals, research material and textbooks in the library when they were done reading them. There I found most of the in-depth material concerning the body's metabolic processes and nutritional data. Having access to a fair number of physicians who, like me, were temporary guests of the USA helped me immensely in this effort as well.

When I was inside, I devoted endless hours to learn the proper way to train. That training was not only about moving heavy iron and increasing my heart rate. It was also becoming knowledgeable in which were the proper foods and nutrients that would contribute to my best performance in the gym. Gone were the days of chips and chocolate. Although they were available in commissary, I totally eliminated them from my diet. I was strict in not only what I ate but how much I ate because that would affect my workouts as well as my general feeling of wellness.

As I continued to train, guys would approach me with pleas to train them at the weight pile and to learn proper nutrition. By this point in my life, I was so into training and conditioning that I wanted to take it to another level. I enrolled in an intensive 6-month course with International Sports Sciences Association (ISSA) the premier fitness institution in the country and became Certified as a personal trainer.

Cheat Days

There is a thought among athletes and serious weightlifters that a day should be set aside weekly to eat whatever you desire. We're not talking about "pigging out" with a 6,000-calorie day (although there are many athletes that consume and burn this amount of calories) but simply to satisfy a craving, enjoy a favorite food or just eating whatever you desire.

Called "cheat days," this is the day that Oreos, chips, pizza, soda and the like won't leave you feeling guilty when you've finished eating them.

Many power lifters will enjoy a cheat day during the week as opposed to a weekend day. The reasoning behind this is because temptation beckons on a weekend. A cheat day can easily become a cheat weekend. Unless you're in the middle of a weight-loss cycle, I do recommend you include a cheat day in your diet. Whatever day you make your cheat day, try to schedule it before your work-set day. Although the body can eliminate the bad stuff within days while eating "clean" the other six, you'll be helping your body to burn off those calories more efficiently with a work-set – the day of the week you lift heavy weights - the following day. Adding cardio work will enhance this process.

In prison, those of us who were strict with their workouts were also focused on eating right. Many of us would schedule our cheat day around our visits. Behind the fence, visiting days are Saturday and Sunday, and it was then that I'd enjoy the foods (if you can call vending machine food enjoyable) I'd normally not have access to, as well as the sugary drinks I otherwise never consumed. Since most of my family and close friends lived a considerable distance from the prison, my cheat days were limited to a day, possibly two, a month. Fortunately, my son Guy lived in Pennsylvania — in Gettysburg actually, owing to his involvement in historical documentaries and movies. Being about an hour and a half away, Guy was able to visit when he wasn't working, however there sometimes were months when I would not have a visit, so I just stuck to my schedule of eating clean.

Chapter 3

Eat your food as your medicines. Otherwise you have to eat medicines as your food

- Steve Jobs

In the last chapter, we talked about the ways in which you can consume your meals and the affects each of those diets has on your body. Now, let's discuss the kinds of foods you put into your body.

Eating in prison is a learned experience. By that I mean *you learn to eat* what you're served, or you don't eat! You are not given the opportunity to take anything more than you're served which is one scoop of this and one scoop of that. Your tray, a small plastic affair, is fitted with four small partitions and one, a bit larger, for the main dish and a spork to eat it with. The food is served cafeteria style and the facility had a nasty habit of serving expired (usually kept in the freezer but many times not) food. Sometimes the food expired years before.

One of my (many) disappointments in prison was the absence of fresh vegetables and the availability of greens for salad. Once or twice a week lettuce was put out in a plastic bin for salads. I recall in the late fall and early winter of 2018 walking into the Chow Hall and discovering Romaine lettuce in place of the Iceberg lettuce we were usually served.

44

Every day for about a week a fresh bin of Romaine lettuce sat chilling on ice for our "enjoyment." A few of those days I opted to eat only those delicious fresh, flavorful, crisp green leaves. The following week while watching the evening news we learned the reason for our bountiful supply of Romaine: it was being discarded throughout the country due to it possibly being contaminated with E. Coli bacteria! Instead of the dumpster, the local grocery stores 'donated' and the prison 'gratefully accepted' this generosity for their criminal charges. Once that cat was out of the bag, none of us ate the Romaine again. Soon after it disappeared from the food line altogether.

You now know that the body burns energy from the food you eat if you allow enough time between meals. If you give your body twelve hours (at least) between the day's last meal and the first meal of the next day, it has the opportunity to properly transmute the food. If you can space sixteen hours (as in the 16:8 diet) between these meals, that is significantly better.

However, it is also important to be mindful of how we consume each meal. The body digests different sources of nutrition in different cycles. Some food remains in the stomach anywhere from two to five hours, while liquids and small particles of food begin to digest almost immediately. To help your body digest more efficiently and more quickly chew your food thoroughly. Poor mastication overworks your digestive system not only causing indigestion but resulting in the retention of food for a longer period of time. Mindfully practice chewing your food at least thirty times. Within ten days you will notice a positive difference in your digestive system.

Human beings enjoy eating. To constantly starve ourselves is not practical nor in any way enjoyable. Fasting has a place in our lives but only if it's done with forethought and common sense. In the long run fasting is not a practical solution or a long-term remedy. And done incorrectly, it can have negative effects on your health.

Measuring Your Portions

Counting calories can be time consuming, however we know that what we eat affects our bodies in many ways. There is also another challenge with counting calories: It is not totally accurate! There can be differences in the quality of the food, laboratory errors, incorrect labeling as well as preparation. The USDA's nutritional database can also be off by as much as 25 percent! How, then, given this information can we control those calories? Actually, the answer is in your own hands!

To determine your protein intake, use your palm. To determine your vegetable portion, use your fist. Your cupped hand will determine your carbohydrate portion and to determine your fat portion use your thumb.

Our hands are scaled to each of us — bigger people need more food and, of course, smaller people need less food. We can control calories by controlling portions. If you take a look at your hands right now you may be surprised at the portion size they would indicate. This method will provide a reasonable amount of each macronutrient (carbs, protein, and fat present in the foods) as well as nutrients found in produce. If you were to eat four meals a day (yes four!) this is what would be a great starting point:

Men:

Two palms of protein-dense foods.

Two fists of vegetables.

Two cupped handfuls of carb-dense foods.

Two thumbs of fat-dense foods.

Women:

One palm of protein-dense foods.

One fist of vegetables.

One cupped handfuls of carb-dense foods.

One thumb of fat-dense foods.[3]

As I continued to carefully observe and control the foods I ate, along with my workouts, I decided that, although a good weight for me was 205 pounds, my ideal weight would be 200. Anything significantly less than that would bring back that gaunt appearance I definitely did not want. Additionally, muscle weighs more than fat and that muscle weight needed to be factored in also. Although I was losing weight, I was continuing to put more weight on the bar as well as increase the reps which continued to inspire me. Finally, having made the decision to allow myself a few lee-way pounds just in case, on October 6, 2019 — just over fourteen weeks later — I achieved my goal of 197 pounds.

Eating is a habit. Eating "good" food is a pleasure. Eating between meals however is generally done out of boredom. Whether you're sitting in front of a TV screen or writing a letter inside of a jail cell, your mind can wander, and food is usually what it focuses on. Sweet, salty, or crunchy are the usual cravings. Most times, these are empty calories, but they also become somewhat difficult to stop eating once you start. Try eating just two potato chips.

In order to satisfy a craving and not pay extra calories, replace that snack with something appetizing and gratifying. Green vegetables are an excellent way to achieve both goals. Celery sticks are quick and easy to get at. "Easy to get at" is important because when you want to reach for the snack, convenience is of paramount concern. One cup of chopped celery is just sixteen calories. Try dipping celery sticks into a small cup of vegetable oil with a pinch of salt and pepper included. It will add a few more calories but the flavor is greatly enhanced. You can also try putting peanut butter on a celery stick. Doing so will not only flatter the taste of the celery but add protein as well. Two tablespoons of peanut butter will add 190 calories but will also provide seven grams of protein. It was a very rare treat when I could get my hands on a stalk of fresh celery in the big house, but it was then that I realized how much I took for granted on the street.

Green beans are another option. Parboil or steam them (steaming is better though as doing so will retain more nutrients as well as flavor) and refrigerate them overnight. Before you eat them the next day mix in a few tablespoons of extra-virgin olive oil, vinegar and a pinch of sea salt for a totally guilt-free snack. For our purposes here it's not necessary to break down meals and specific recipes, however, let's look at what foundationally is necessary lose fat and gain muscle.

To begin, multiply your present body weight by twelve. This number will determine the number of calories you want to consume to maintain your current weight. For example, your current weight is 230 pounds therefore your daily calorie intake should be no more than 2,760 calories.

But now let's suppose that you would like to bring your weight down to 200 pounds. You would want to consume no more than 2,400 calories a day. In order to take maximum advantage of your weightlifting routine, you should begin consuming protein. There are a few schools of thought on protein ingestion that you may be familiar with but with full disclosure in mind let's look at a few of them here.

For someone over the age of forty, protein consumption significantly augments muscle growth. Simply put, when we lift weights, we put a substantial amount of stress on the targeted muscle. This stress causes minute damage to the muscle tissue, which then produces new proteins in order to heal.

Some studies suggest .74 grams of protein per pound of body weight. A 230-pound man would therefore require 170 grams per day. Other studies suggest one and a half grams of protein for each pound of body weight for heavy lifters. Federal guidelines suggest fifty-six grams of protein a day for men and forty-six grams for women. These numbers were consistent with the menu fed to those of us in prison. I was able to supplant this somewhat by drinking skim milk throughout the day as well as with a few of the higher-protein items such as peanut butter, chicken breast, and a low-grade protein powder, all which were available at the commissary once a week. I managed to ingest about 100 grams of protein at most, but not every day, which was half of what I really needed but just enough given my circumstances.

In any event, the general consensus is 1 gram of protein per pound per day as the most efficient for the body of someone weightlifting or athletic. As noted earlier, proteins, carbohydrates and fats are macronutrients that someone should watch closely if they are serious about their nutrition and achieving optional health and athleticism. Let's look at the example of a 230-pound man:

A 230-pound man should eat 230 grams of protein per day. Thirty percent of his daily calories should come from fat. A 230-pound man should consume 828 calories of fat daily. It is easier to count in grams, though. So, since a gram of fat contains nine calories, divide 828 by nine which will give you ninety-two grams of fat.

Proteins and carbs contain four calories per grams so our 230-pound guy will be ingesting 920 calories of protein daily (230 pounds of weight/grams x four calories).

The remaining calories will come from carbohydrates. The calculations for our guy would look like this:

2,760 calories

- 828 calories from fat

- 920 calories from protein

1,012 calories from carbs

Converting carbohydrates and protein into grams gives us 230 grams of protein and 253 grams of carbs (920 divided by four equals 230 grams of protein; 1012 divided by four equals 253 grams of carbohydrates).

If your goal is to drop weight, use all of the calculations above to determine your goal numbers. For example, your current weight is, as above, 230 pounds but your goal is 180 pounds you would now consume 2,160 calories per day (180 x 12) 648 calories of fat, 720 calories of protein and 792 calories of carbohydrates. You can plug in any number you choose using these calculations.

The Healthiest Options

Some years back there was a campaign toward limiting or eliminating meat, especially beef, from our diet. Numerous studies have shown that consuming meat, especially high-fat content meat at every meal can lead to diabetes, heart disease, obesity, and a propensity for contracting cancer.

Keep in mind however that our pre-historic ancestors flourished by consuming animal flesh. Our teeth bear testimony to this. Human beings possess teeth for gripping, ripping, and tearing. We possess two upper and two lower teeth called incisors and two more upper and lower teeth called canines.

Be conscious of your meat consumption and be strict with your general nutrition by consuming extra lean cuts of beef as well as skinless poultry or fish. A three-ounce boneless and skinless chicken breast would yield 110 calories and twenty-five grams of protein. A three-ounce cut of wild Atlantic salmon would have 153 calories and twenty-one grams of protein. Meanwhile a six-ounce filet mignon would provide thirty grams of protein and 490 calories.[4]

Starches such as rice, potatoes, and sweet potatoes would be healthy choices to go for your carbs, and a few pieces of fruit per day to satisfy a sweet tooth. Keep in mind that extra fructose (the soluble sugar found in fruit juices and honey) can slow the fat burning process and promotes fat storage. Your liver (where bile is secreted as well as being the center of your metabolic activity) can effectively process only a limited amount of glycogen and you should be mindful of this when choosing foods.

Water intake, like sleep, is a necessary part of your life. When a person is focused on weight loss, drinking water can help to take the edge off-of hunger pangs. Water causes the brain to create electrical energy resulting in the production of testosterone, nerve activation and alertness. It keeps the muscles strong as well as thinning the blood which in turn assists the liver to properly filter harmful substances such as germs, pollutants and alcohol from your body. Water causes the small intestines to circulate fluids throughout the body delivering amino acids (used by the body's cells to build proteins) fats and sugars, all necessary for the cells to function properly. It can also prevent overly dry skin.

One gallon of water — 128 ounces or about ten, ten-ounce glasses of water — spaced out throughout the day will help you stay hydrated. You should be aware that coffee, tea, juices, and milk contain water which can help with hydration.

It may seem surprising, but the body *absorbs* hydration easier than drinking fluids. When foods hold a high percentage of water, they help a person by feeling full. Foods like cucumbers, watermelon, tomatoes, spicy peppers, cantaloupe, and honeydew can contain up to 90 percent water, as do eggplant and kiwi. Research has offered that it may be better to eat water instead of drinking it!

Each of our bodies are genetically unique to us and as such our way of digesting fluids and foods is also. Generally stated however, some foods can remain in the stomach for a few hours while others can remain for up to five hours. Liquids and small particles of food begin to digest almost immediately but putting an all-out effort into any workout after you've eaten is counterproductive as we've seen.

In the end, when it's all been said and done, what matters most is how serious you are in losing weight, achieving health and getting strong — and maintaining those objectives once you achieve them. You, luckily, do not need to be on guard for a bodily assault from a street thug in a prison yard, but you want to be able to prevent heart disease, stave off cancer if possible, and live a full and energy-filled life.

SUPPLEMENTS

We've discussed the importance of good nutrition, various types of fasts and the cogent supposition regarding cellular restoration. To effectively assist your goal of getting bigger, stronger and leaner the addition of a solid supplement plan will not only support your efforts to achieve those goals but will intensify the results significantly.

Protein supplements are a product that most serious weightlifters are familiar with and use frequently. The body uses protein to help repair cells as well as to create new cells. Interestingly, when water is taken out of the equation, 15 to 20 percent of body weight is protein, but unlike carbohydrates and fat, it is not stored in the body. For someone who is a serious lifter as well as for people over forty, extra protein is essential.

In the Bureau of Prisons (BOP) system, protein supplements — at least quality protein supplements, were not available. At my last bid — the word "bid," by the way, can refer to a specific prison location, the amount of time given or the last time a person was in prison (sadly there are many who are multiple repeaters) — there was what they called a "Health Shake" available at the commissary. This formula provided twenty-four grams of protein but was loaded with sugar, carbs, fats, and sodium. It was extremely expensive as well. As we'll discuss in a minute, all protein supplements are *not* the same, and it is prudent to become informed before purchasing any.

Muscle consists mostly of protein and lifting weights stresses the muscle tissue causing minute damage to that tissue. In order to heal, that damage is what initiates new protein. The muscle will also devour any excess protein traveling throughout the bloodstream. This effect necessitates a weight trainee to not only ingest enough food but to eat cleanly. Research has shown that not doing so will cause lean muscle *loss*.

Supplements are foundational for anyone looking to become healthier but is especially so for someone whose goal is to increase strength and get lean. The following are a few of the basic supplements to assist you in achieving this.

WHEY PROTEIN

Whey protein is what's known as a soluble substance meaning it dissolves in liquid. Twenty percent of the protein found in milk is whey. It is the best-selling protein powder on the market due to its ability to build lean muscle. Although whey protein digests fairly quickly, it is best not taken immediately before lifting. The challenge of drinking anything immediately prior to a workout (water being the exception) is due to the large amount of blood required with the digestive process. When the blood is tied up in digestion cramping can develop as well as improperly breaking down other chemicals in the body. Drinking whey protein delivers its amino acids (nitrogen-containing acids used by the body's cells to build protein) within sixty to ninety minutes so ingesting this protein an hour or two before lifting is the best option.

You may have heard the term *branched-chained amino acids* (usually referred to as BCAA's) in the past and not quite known what they are or the importance they play in muscle development. The acids L-Leucine, L-Isoleucine and L-Valine make up BCAAs. BCAAs comprise 35 percent of muscle tissue and stimulates the production of insulin. During highly intense training BCAAs are burned as fuel and at the end of long-distance events when the body recruit's protein for as ' much as 20 percent of the energy needed to endure. [5]

We must also consider the contrast between various grades of whey protein. Whey is the liquid substance that remains from the cheese making process. Once this is separated and dried it is put forth as Whey Protein Concentrate. This is then filtered but that filtration process allows for a wide range of protein quality.

Whey Protein Concentrate 80 percent is considered the gold standard while Whey Protein Concentrate 30 percent is considered the lowest. The gradings of whey protein will vary between the two.

As of this writing the FDA does not require manufacturers to disclose the grade of protein, but you can contact the protein company and ask for a composition grade of their Whey Protein Concentrate that is NON-GMO (Non-Genetically Modified Corn, used as a usual protein additive), free of growth hormones, is organic and has no artificial flavors, dyes, or ingredients.

CASEIN

Unlike whey protein which digests fairly quickly, casein protein is very slow to digest.

Casein can take as long as seven hours to deliver all its amino acids to the muscles. Because of this slower delivery it's recommended that casein be ingested prior to bedtime. Casein makes up the remaining 80 percent of milk's primary type of protein, however cottage cheese or Greek yogurt are good choices to ingest before going to bed. These are great sources of casein, but you could also drink it in a protein shake as well. Studies have shown that adding Casein to whey protein after working out can increase muscle growth beyond what's likely with whey protein on its own.

CREATINE

When I was lifting in the '90s another supplement that was beginning to get a lot of attention was creatine. Since that time, creatine has become one of the most researched supplements and has been found to be a very effective one. Research confirmed that about ten pounds of muscle mass could be added to the guy who lifts and an additional 10 percent increase — or more — in muscle strength.

Creatine is absorbed by the muscle cells which in turn uses it as an enhancement to fuel muscle contractions during a workout. This results in more reps completed and increases in muscle strength and size. As a pre-workout amino acid, creatine can be taken just prior to lifting as its ingested with water only and dissolves into the water so cramping should not be an issue.

Behind the walls and razor wire you learn to make do as I wrote earlier but never doubt for a moment that you can't get your hands on what's considered "contraband" by the prison authorities. Cell phones, cigarettes, food, drugs, steroids, and "stuff" you couldn't imagine. For the right price, a severe lack of judgement, and the possibility of harsh penalties if caught, you can obtain most anything.

Some of the jailhouse strong men were unbelievably bulked up and cut. No matter how much fish and chicken you eat, you can't get that chiseled on these alone. Not in a prison yard, at least. A case in point:

One of the half-witted he-men on the compound juiced up regularly, and, like any addiction, couldn't get off the merry-go-round. One day, after injecting the usual dose of phony-muscle formula in his butt he began howling like a banshee. Hiding the steroids somewhere on the compound, he neglected to allow his secret nectar to thaw out to room temperature, causing the fluid to congeal under the skin forming a sizable knot. One of his workout buddies, according to a guy who witnessed the performance, kindly massaged his backside trying to dissipate the phony fluid. We were still rolling our eyes about it when I left prison. What a sight that must have been, and I'm glad I missed it!

Eating clean, eating on a regular schedule, and supplementing your diet with a solid supplement plan — along with a dedicated and consistent training program will enhance your capability to build a body of size, flexibility, and endurance.

SLEEP

While not directly related to our food consumption, sleep is important to mention in a chapter all about what we put into our bodies. When we put in rest, along with a healthy diet and hard physical work, we get good results out of it. The importance of adequate sleep cannot possibility be overstated if you are serious about your health, as well as weight and cardio training.

There are two states of sleep: REM (rapid eye movement) and non-REM. Most of our sleep time is spent in the non-REM state, however when we enter the REM state our learning, reasoning, and emotions are nourished. Amazingly brain waves are similar during REM as they are for a wide- awake person!

Sleep also has been found to 'brand' memories of those events we've recently encountered into our brain. Unfortunately, our culture has been associating sleep or rest time with laziness and lack of motivation for many years, however a new generation of forward thinkers and enlightened folks have been bringing to public view the creativity and work ethic provided for by a well-rested individual. For our purpose though, we need to embrace the restorative benefits available through sleep.

Unlike free men, many convicts are not only able to get a full nights' sleep but are able to take naps during the day. There is usually thirty to sixty minutes after lunch for an inmate to get a few minutes of sleep before they need to report back to work. These rest breaks were great for the guys lifting heavy. Now before you become too resentful of what you've just read, please consider the following: There is not a con alive who wouldn't want to trade places with you! Keep in mind that the least of your worries is being pummeled with a padlock-in-a-sock while you're sleeping or being beaten by a group of gangbangers while your eyes are tightly shut. It happens. On the block you quickly learn to grow eyes in the back of your head.

In lock-up, inmates are on a schedule — something to perhaps emulate if getting prison-strong is a goal. Going to sleep at the same time and waking up at a regular, set time will lend itself well to the body's circadian rhythm. The circadian rhythm is the twenty-four-hour interval of biological activity and by setting specific times to retire for the night and waking in the morning you will, after a few weeks, adapt which will allow your body to take full positive advantage of a new way of living.

If possible, take a twenty- to thirty-minute nap mid-afternoon. This is the time the circadian rhythm lowers the body's energy level. The body recovers during sleep and most of its natural growth hormones is produced during REM sleep. When a person is sleep-deprived they crave sugar-filled foods which as we've seen can have adverse cellular effects on the body.

A study recently conducted by the University of Chicago Medical School addressed the importance of a full night's sleep.

Two control groups which the university organized were put on a calorie-restricted diet with one of the groups getting a full night's sleep but not the other. While both groups lost the same amount of weight, the group who were sleep-deprived had less fat loss by 25 percent!

A minimum amount of seven hours of uninterrupted sleep is recommended. Eight hours would be better. Avoid taking sleeping pills as the sleep they induce lacks the recuperation power the body depends on. Sleeping less than six hours is likely to deplete muscle if you are restricting calories. Your gains in the weight room will be negligible, if any at all, with less than six hours of sleep. Additionally, you may set yourself up for other conditions such as hypertension and diabetes. Lastly, avoid big meals within four hours of going to sleep as the digestion process will interfere with the body's relaxation manner.

Chapter 4

You don't find will power – you create it

Anonymous

When I trudged into prison in 2011, I committed myself to taking weight off my 6 foot frame. And I did—fat *and* muscle mass. When I was transferred to the prison in Northeast Pennsylvania, Schuylkill. I realized just what I had done to myself. By that point, I was a skeletal looking 174 lbs.!

When someone enters prison, as a new inmate or one that's been transferred from another facility, they are stripped-searched, fingerprinted and photographed. I guess that a person doesn't notice their appearance day to day (at least not behind bars), but when I saw my photo at Schuylkill that day, I was shocked! I mean a literal jolt of " electricity" hit me in the stomach. I looked appalling! It was if I walked out of a dungeon (which I suppose was fitting given the circumstances).

Later that day as I was unpacking my meager possessions, I noticed my skin. It hung, flowed really from my biceps. I was stunned. I was embarrassed, and I silently vowed I would do something about it. I began the very next day.

Eventually, as the months turned into years at Schuylkill, I got stronger, but I also gained weight. After a few years of lifting and eating I topped out at 227 — more than fifty pounds from when I reported to Schuylkill.

Since I was making significant gains at the weight pile by then (the skin now firm and taut), I developed a long-range plan. I would grow as strong as I could then regulate myself with a program designed to keep the muscle but loose the fat.

For a few years I hovered between 227 and 215 pounds, but the average always seemed to be 221 — my high school graduation weight. I made up my mind to take off the pounds. I was no longer fat, but my goal now was strong *and* lean.

By the summer of 2019, I knew that my time in prison would be winding down, I began to think deeply about my life once I left the walls, razor wire and the bars behind. I had struggled with so much since that spring day in 2008 when the United States came calling (let alone what my company's investors had also endured) and among those matters was the knowledge of what physically could happen when I was to return to the life of the living. I knew of guys that left prison and ate "normally" again and proceeded to pack on pounds. I read of one guy who gained 60 pounds within three months! If you're not mindful of your weight it can happen quickly. With that thought in mind I decided to drop my weight again.

From my past experience of losing so many pounds, I decided that a good weight for my six-foot frame, accounting for a body with muscle, would be 205. I began this regimen on June 27, 2019 at 220 pounds. I decided to weigh myself daily. Doing so, for me, would give me the opportunity to catch myself quickly and do something about it before gaining any weight would get out of hand. Nothing was more frustrating than to put on an extra pound or two despite being strict. But my daily weigh-in allowed me to catch it quickly and adjust for it. XX

In Chapter 1 we talked about the importance of cardio to lose weight. In Chapters 2 and 3, we talked about the most effective and efficient way to fuel your body. Now let's dive into the exciting stuff: weightlifting and strength training.

CORE STRENGTH

True strength is accomplished when every part of the body works in concert. We're familiar with the body types of a bulked-up guy as well as the guy who's dedicated to running or into cardio fitness training. Each of these accomplishments took dedication and consistency to achieve, however to be strong, conditioned, *and* toned, we need to engage all the different parts of the body in unison. This is known as physical integration.

To correctly train our bodies, we need to begin at the foundation of our body — the core. This, by the way, holds true when building a business. Both must begin at the foundation. Whether you are beginning a training program for the first time or are an experienced lifter or cardio enthusiast if your core strength is lacking, you may not reach your maximum physical potential.

The expression "core strength" is a fairly new idiom. According to the "Corpus of Historical American English" the term "core strength" didn't appear in everyday use until 1997, yet core strength is an attribute that has been part of the human race since man's appearance on Earth.

In order to survive in a hostile world our prehistoric ancestors had to rely on gut instinct, cognitive thinking and inner muscular endurance. He had to be able to throw a spear, wield a club, climb a tree, outrun a predator, or stand and fight. (Sounds a bit like prison!) These early forebears of ours needed to develop a strong core and maintain that strength knowing their very lives depended on doing so.

When someone thinks of the body's core, they consider the abdominals as that spot and while our midsection is part of the core, there are more muscles involved. Although some trainers argue that nearly every muscle in the body is part of the core, identifying and then working those muscles located between the fifth rib and the sitting bones, will develop the foundation in which to achieve a sturdy muscular physique.

In order to perform cardio training as well as weightlifting the spine must be capable of supporting the force placed upon it. Acquiring and maintaining a strong core can, simply put, stabilize the spine and assist in taking weight off of it.

For years prior to my legal challenges, I frequently experienced back pain. More often than not, the pains were severe. These muscle spasms resulted in recurring visits to the chiropractor. When I was lifting heavy, especially squatting when I was younger, I would go in for a back adjustment a few times a month due to the downward pressure on my spine. Although I was strong, my core was weak. This went on for years.

After languishing in prison for a few years I discovered the secret to strengthening my back. And, it turned out, the rest of my midsection. The midsection of the body includes the anterior and posterior —the front and the back- and there are specific exercises and moves that focus specifically on the muscles located there. These exercises include planks, side planks, crunches, and leg raises. Personally, once I became adapt with these moves, I continued to seek out additional methods that would increase the strength of my core. I found the means to do so through yoga.

Yoga has the ability to build core strength not only on a physical and emotional level, but a spiritual one as well. Let me state here: As a Christian I find no conflict between practicing yoga and my faith. There are no chants, prayers, or mantras involved in yogic moves. There are no idols that are worshipped through yoga, however a deep piety (for want of a better word) that came from interconnectedness between my body and soul and God was something that I found exhilarating.

Even though I am no expert, performing nearly twenty yogic poses (there are dozens) assisted me in developing a full range of motion that helped my sense of balance as well as my strength while lessening the risk of injury to my muscles. As my core became stronger my other workouts became more effective.

There are a variety of exercises to help develop your core. Whether you're doing time for breaking and entering or spending time in a hotel room between company break-out sessions, working on your core strength is not complicated. There are no machines or equipment needed. Similar to body weight exercises, which we'll discuss in a bit, core exercises require only determination, commitment, and consistency.

Before we leave the topic of core strength, allow me to share the following.....

In prison, loneliness is prevalent, even though it would not seem possible as you are rarely alone. But loneliness, like happiness, comes from within. On the life outside you have family, friends, and acquaintances to share concerns as well as successes, with. You ask for opinions as well as advice and, depending on the strength of the relationship, you may or may not take that guidance. In prison, you learn to never trust anyone. Most cons have their own agenda and sharing personal issues as well as information is not something usually done. That said you may meet that one, or if you're really blessed, a handful out of the thousands of inmates you come in contact with. I had one such blessing. I made a few close acquaintances and for that I am thankful, but Dave was that one I could and did share my goals, ideas, and dreams with.

Shortly after my transfer to Schuylkill, I began to notice a narrowing of vision in my left eye. What began subtly after a few days became terrifying. Thankfully one of the medical staff saw the seriousness of my condition and sent me to an outside eye-specialist where emergency surgery for a detached retina was performed.

Our God works in mighty and unexpected ways.......Let me explain.

I had been to the medical office several times prior concerning my deepening eye problem. The day before I went again and once again was blown off. "Ahhhh, come back tomorrow....". I did. Miraculously, there sat a guy alone in the office, who I had never seen before. Without hesitation, he picked up the phone and had me immediately rushed to an eye specialist on the outside. Afterward, the doctor told me I had been within hours of losing the sight in that eye permanently. Had it not been for a 'chance' meeting with someone I never saw prior.............

Returning, I was helpless. Dave took it upon himself to nurse me back to health. Leaving his bunk on another floor in the middle of the night, Dave put the many drops needed to aid in restoring my sight. He did this for weeks. Jesus said, "As you did it to the least of My brothers you did it to Me." Dave lived those words.

But each of us — incarcerated or free — are not immune from life's problems and challenges. Developing your inner fortitude is a goal that can be achieved with strength development. If you have ever lost your job, had true financial hardship, lost a loved one or had someone you adored walk out on you, you know that strong shoulders, sculpted abs or a chiseled physique aren't what carry's you through. What does is strength of heart, mental, and emotional toughness and spiritual fortitude.

Without these, prison is nearly impossible to navigate, but more importantly these attributes determine character, confidence, understanding, and resoluteness in the free world.

BODY WEIGHT EXERCISES

Staying in one piece in federal prison is dependent on being prepared. Preparation means you assess the situation, decide what steps you'll need to take to handle a possible future, and then put that plan into action. You pick a workout routine and although you may need to change it around and ramp it up you know that you are becoming a one-man army.

You never forget that you're living with guys with crazy eyes, shaved heads, muscular and powerful frames and bad attitudes.

Some have gentle names like T', M, Q, Daylight, Midnight, Fat Man, or Face. My prison nom-de-guerre was Gino. Others were known by Beast, Gangster, and Murder, among others. Very, very few were guys to mess with. Shanks and shives (knives to you), razor blades, and padlocks-in-a-sock are all prohibited, very lethal, and ever-present. It is critical to get jacked quickly even if free weights aren't available.

My first few years in prison were one's of adjustment — putting my head around a thirteen-year sentence overpowered my very being. Realizing that despite my hopes and dreams of seeing home again anytime soon, all that I had left to cling to were my memories. Memories and visions that were powerful enough to almost touch - the softness of my wife's skin, her eyes when she would look at me. The love we shared between us. The memories of the smiles she would give me that caused me to smile even in all the darkness surrounding me. It was the knowledge that eventually I would be back to where things made sense. Where I could dream real dreams again. Where, once more, I could hold her in my arms, share Sunday dinner with her, with our children and soon grandchildren......

But this was now, and the only thing left to do, the only things I *could* control, were to take command of my mind and my body. With the determination of making this bitter experience worth something, I seized my fate by the trachea and made it happen.

Those first two years were my initiation to prison. I went about allowing, forcing really, my attitude, my personality, and my character to adjust. To become strong enough to survive.

I was fortunate, blessed really, to have those few "guardian angels" watching my back. Those brother Italians who looked out for me while I learned the rules of prison and, as I wrote earlier, nobody messed with them. But what I learned I had to learn on my own and by my third year on the compound I was learning and working hard.

At Elkton, where I began my sentence, free weights were not available. It was just as well, because my main focus as I wrote, was in losing weight and gaining endurance. I succeeded, but I also began doing body weight exercises. Slowly at first, but after my permanent transfer to Schuylkill, I brought it up another level. A much higher level.

As an inmate, you learn to be creative in most anything thrown at you. Whether it's cooking or reacting to a wise mouth, organizing a locker with cracker boxes as a storage space or standing your ground — you get it done. It's basic training for living a basic existence.

Your time out of the block is strictly limited as well as strictly monitored. Lockdowns happen just as you're heading to the weight pile. The yard gets shutdown just as you're starting your first set. Fog sets in for the morning so a recall back to your block is announced, messing up your cardio training or the rec yard is locked down for weeks because some joker left his steroid syringes under the mat in the lifting area which results in mass punishment. All of these obstacles cause a serious crimp in your training.

The con doesn't let minor annoyances like these prevent his progress of packing on muscle however, most guys use body weight training during times like to these. Whether it's a cell or a cubicle, the warrior uses compound exercises to build strong shoulders, massive quads, and crushing grips.

If weights are available these should be the first choice in your training routine. However, there are those instances when weights are not accessible and when that happens body weight moves can abet your training. The body has three primary areas: the lower torso, the upper torso, and the head. The lower torso, where the majority of muscles are located accounts for about 65 percent of body weight. The upper torso where the vital organs reside makes up about 30 percent of body weight and the head the remaining 5 percent. Although this is a general rule of thumb you get the idea.

Body weight exercises generally include push-ups, burpees, jumping jacks, crunches, body squats, dips, chin ups or pull-ups, and leg raises. There are a variety of performance styles when using some of these moves during training and we'll be reviewing them later.

On any given day there seems to be an endless parade of products designed to enhance a man's libido. The television network executives know their demographic — guys who want to get strong, look good, and score with women. "Try this formula for thirty days, and you'll see the difference!" Sounds easy enough. The problem is, however, it will take a great deal of effort to realistically achieve these goals. Your money is better spent for a gym membership.

Testosterone levels in most guys on the outside world can usually not compare to a guy in lockdown. Most cons have a higher-than-average testosterone level which displays itself with higher-than-average aggressiveness and violent tendencies. The common criminal exhibits high-risk behavior, a high degree of energy and a propensity to "take care of business now!" Take the average Joe who used his brain to get ahead in the free world and lock him up with truly bad boys and watch what happens. He either becomes very "compliant" or he decides to man up. Quickly.

In prison, there is a brutish subculture who dispense with words and act out with fists. Or worse. It's the mindset of the barbarian and what ratchets up the belligerent and combative behavior is the lack of female companionship. Although common in many state facilities conjugal visits are not allowed in the Federal Bureau of Prisons. One begins to wonder how many marriages, how many families would be saved if there were. Looking back, I suppose this is another opportunity to punish someone, and this in a very personal and soul-crushing way.

The pent-up pugnacity that a man feels behind bars must by nature have an outlet. Workouts do more than get a guy pumped. They release a lot of tension and pent-up frustrations. Consequently, the guy behind bars attacks the weight pile with a vengeance. To many of them, it's their primary goal, the highlight of an otherwise depressing and monotonous existence. I know it became mine.

By the time I was transferred to Schuylkill, ten years had passed since I last lifted seriously or even picked up an Olympic bar. I knew that I needed to set a daily schedule to begin working out, and once I did, I began working with an empty bar to get my form and technique back.

Those few weeks were a wake-up call. Tears rolled down my face (they must have thought it was sweat!) as I struggled to lift even the lightest of weights. Miraculously I didn't get thrown out of the weight pit with my performance. Maybe they felt sorry for me. I never knew. What I could easily lift or press in 2003 now felt like 1,000 pounds. Fortunately, muscle has memory so with focus, commitment, and consistency I began to make progress. Slowly but steadily.

As you begin your journey, or if you've been away from lifting for a while and just getting back into it again, use caution and common sense. *Start light.* It is wise to have a goal in mind when you decide to begin weight training. This goal should be specific but realistic. A certified fitness trainer, for instance, would work with you by putting together definite objectives, and they'll construct, teach, and motivate you to achieve those goals. Over time, you will begin to notice how your body is responding to weight training by improving strength and muscle size. This is known as *neural adaption* which is the responsiveness of the sensory system to a constant stimulus — in this case, lifting weights.

As the years at Schuylkill went by, I began training guys in the same way my buddy John trained me so many years before —with a broomstick and with an empty bar. This is the best way to learn. Once your form is in place you begin adding weight.

When you are locked in a cage, you hear a lot of talk. A lot of jive. But at a prison weight pit, you also hear about exercises that you've never come across before. You see guys who've been down ten, fifteen, twenty-five years and more with an attitude of leaving nothing on the table.

Personally, I began to push myself to limits I could never have imagined. I guess when you're locked up for years, your head starts playing with you. Simply put: I beat up my body. It was as if I dared my age to stop me. It didn't. With that mindset it is important to lift correctly—correct form and correct technique.

In prison you avoid getting hurt, but you do *everything* to avoid getting injured. A trip to medical where if an injury is categorized as serious can sideline a man for months due to a mandatory "medical idle". If the injury is traced back to the weight room, guys have been known to get dragged out of the weight room to another area of the prison, you can be indefinitely banned from going back. If an injury was due to a fight at the weight pit, the weights may be permanently removed.

I recall a pushing match that very quickly escalated to plates about to be used as weapons. By this point, I had not only been at Schuylkill for a few years but behind the fence as well, so I had that "cred" I talked about earlier. Although I made it my habit to keep out of other people's business, I stepped between the two fighters knowing that the weights would be taken away if one of their foreheads were to be caved in. Cool heads prevailed, and they went their separate ways.

GENETICS

As I was working out in the weight pile one day, I noticed a young black guy (In prison you are referred to as a white guy, a black guy, or a Spanish guy) who had just joined us a few days before, walk over to a flat bench and start doing reps. Now just walking over to the weight pit is not really done, you must be invited as I've related, but this kid (he was probably twenty-five or so) grabbed a straight (Olympic) bar and started repping 135 pounds like it was an empty bar! No warm-up, no stretching, nothing. The amazing thing however was he was about five-foot-ten-inches tall and 160 pounds soaking wet! I watched in amazement![6]

Genetics does account for the speed of muscle gain, the symmetry of those muscles and physique of the person. The challenge when lifting is knowing what muscles to target, how to train them and ultimately end up with the body form desired.

Bone density, height, eye color, musculature, and so much more are passed on from generation to generation. Although there is nothing you can do about your genetic history, you can specifically focus on weaknesses. Usually there is a body part that is weak, or weaker than the others. The reason is, more often than not, a genetic deficiency.

When most guys walk into a gym (especially if this is their first visit to a gym), they visualize becoming massive. Every guy who works out wants that chiseled-in-marble look but at times it feels so elusive. One of a gym guy's biggest frustrations is watching other guys move more weight than they do.

When a person is massively strong, looking like they belong in a lifting magazine you can be sure that genetics have something to do with that. Motor neuron coordination as well as tendon size gives guys like that a huge advantage over others.

If getting exceptionally strong is a goal of yours plan on working the same body part twice a week. Take a longer pause between sets, three to five minutes at least with each set consisting of two to five heavy-weight reps.

Most people don't train this way. Higher reps, lower weight and shorter rest pauses of forty-five seconds to a minute between sets is the usual routine to get cut. But if building over-the-top strength is important to you, this is the method to use.

Some guys have wide hips which makes the V-tape back difficult to achieve. Difficult but not impossible.

The solution to this genetic dilemma is to concentrate on the upper back. Working your lats and teres major as well as the rhomboids and the teres minor will add width to your back. Exercises like 1-arm dumbbell rows, bent-over barbell rows, and T-bar rows will greatly assist you here but for the red-meat, chin-ups and pull-downs can't be surpassed for adding width to a guy's back.

There is an abundance of material available online that addresses genetic weaknesses and the exercises designed to surmount them. You'll find the exercise that, done properly and consistently, can overcome any of these weaknesses. Training with a partner can usually help you work through sticking points during a lift. Personally, my training was an escape for me, so I preferred to lift by myself. But if I were doing a work-set day - lifting heavy - I made sure others were around just in case.

When you work with another, make certain they can help you if you need it. Called a 'spotter,' this is the person that can hand off a heavy barbell and lift it back up if you're in a hole. This is critical. I recall one of the heavier lifters in the yard having a newbie spot him. This guy was performing incline bench presses. Increasing the weight to 235 pounds, he did his lift-off while relying on his spotter to guide the bar directly above his chest, arms outstretched. Instead, his spotter guided the bar over his stomach! Arms now awkwardly extended and milliseconds from a major injury I jumped up and helped bring the bar back to the rack. Bottom line: Know who you're working with.

If there is a particular area that becomes a sticking point, like if your bench press maxes out at 205, for example, have a spotter assist you on your one rep max. Let's consider that number to be 225 pounds.

With those 225 pounds in mind, perform five sets of three reps with 80 percent of that weight, in this case 180 pounds. Take a few weeks to work up to five sets of five reps then determine after the third week what your one-rep max is and adjust your workout accordingly.

Working your body is a challenge. The body does not like pain, does not want pain, and will do anything to avoid pain. It's those pain receptors that synapse. "Cut it out. This hurts!" they say to your conscious mind. This is where strength of character and strength of heart comes into play. By disciplining yourself to overcome resistance to abusing your body, making it uncomfortable, making it work to do what you want it to do, you will carry over that success to all other areas of your life! You can build on that mindset, that success. Why? Because you will have amazed yourself that you could do it. And if you could do that, you'll know you can do anything that you put your heart and soul into. You'll see.

PHILOSOPHY

Chapter 5

Let the tears of your heart water the seeds of your future....

Count it all joy when you fall into various trials, knowing that the testing of your faith produces patience." 7

These words, taken from the Bible held a very special meaning to me during my trials with the government. Each day during the ordeal brought, it seemed, new challenges to deal with, new obstacles to overcome and new sorrows to manage......

It was in the late fall, those days known as Indian Summer, that time of year when the sun shines dimly and softly. The sky turns a rich and vibrant blue during a Western New York Indian Summer, and as you take in the magnificence it appears gentle and hazy to the eye. The leaves have been painted a brilliant red and an intense shade of gold. It is a warm and inviting time of the year and brings with it the promise of an autumn filled with love and the gratitude of having family surrounding you. It was at that time of year that I traveled southwest from my home in Buffalo, New York.

Instead of the beauty of clear blue skies, that morning was, appropriately for me anyway, dreary and overcast with a light drizzle falling onto the leaf-filled roads. For hours we traveled along the southern shore of Lake Erie towards my ultimate destination a few miles outside of Youngstown, Ohio, to what is known as Federal Correctional Institution Elkton.

With me that day was my best friend, my confidant, and the woman I most cherished in this world: my wife Bethann. My son Geoffrey drove, along with his wife Jen, allowing Bethann and I to cling to each other for our last few hours together in the backseat. My son Guy, an actor, was on location that day and was unable to be with us. My daughter Jenna, involved in Christian Ministry in Kansas City, was not able to make it home in time. It was Jenna who showed me what loving the Lord was about. In short, she was my inspiration.

My stepson Ryan. Leaving him in his formative years, a teenager who would now have to become the man of the house, taking over the responsibilities of someone far older, hurt beyond knowing. Then my beautiful little angel Juliann. Leaving her behind, seeing the teardrops dripping down her face cut into my heart a thousand ways. She was not 'just' my stepdaughter, but part of my soul. I would miss her so much. Looking back to those days, only God in His infinite wisdom knew how I was able to go on without them all.

Finally, and inexorably, we arrived to where the life I knew would end and the life I would forevermore know would begin.

As we walked through those prison doors a sense of power overcame me. Not mine certainly, but the power of an institution, a government that is able to take total control over a person's life. Solid blocks of stone, razor wire — six double-edged rows of it — and a tangible foreboding sense overpowered me.

Trying to remain strong I drew my wife close to me, tears streaming down her beautiful face as I so desperately wanted to impart the feeling of the immense love I had for her, a feeling that would have to last us a decade.

My daughter-in-law Jen who, pregnant with my first grandchild, was every bit my own child, eyes soaked with grief hugged me goodbye.

And Geoffrey, my son who stood by me through every arrow and barb thrown at me and written about me. As I looked deeply into his eyes, I saw the unbelief, the confusion and the realization that only a moment like this could bring forth. I held my boy in my arms, seeing the anguish and pain etched on his face and I was overwhelmed. The realization that it was I who, through naivety and misguidedness, was responsible for this all, was overpowering.

And although not with me physically, the investors of my company WaterMark walked with me into prison that day. They, helpless to do anymore, would have to wait until the day I left prison for the last time. Though they may not have believed it at that time, I was then, am now, and will always be committed to repaying them. And along with God's help, I would.

As I turned away from my family, following one of my new caretakers, I knew I was leaving the life of the living to enter the U.S. Justice Department's version of the living dead. When I entered my housing unit, my heart seemed to stop. I felt as if the oxygen was immediately taken from my lungs as from a vacuum. The noise, the congestion, the total confusion and mayhem overwhelmed my senses. As I made my way to my bunk, with my bed roll, towel, and prison clothes slung over my shoulder, I felt every eye follow my steps throughout the block. "What's this guy's story?" "Where'd he come from?" "What'd he do?" "How easy can I take advantage of this guy?"

I was still a big boy back then. Big but physically weak. Concerned? Absolutely. Like you I heard all the prison stories. The fights, the showers (and the soap), the rapes, the stabbings. Are they true? What do you think?

Every manner of personality is found in lockdown. The murderer, the bank robber, the "made" guys, the gangbangers and the gang leaders. The white-collar guys like me. To say I was scared would be overstating it. But not by much.

There is a testosterone-filled pecking order in prison that I came to find. Near the top of the pyramid were the armed drug dealers. These were the gunslingers, the mavericks who took their lives in their hands every day. Then the average street dealer. Next were the thieves-bank robbers and armored car hijackers, then the white-collar guys like me. Further down, much further down, were what are known as 'cho-mos.' In prison there is nothing lower, nothing worse than the child pornographer. The child molester. The guy who either having, or was about to before he got caught, sex with a child. If there were a more reviled, more reprehensible inmate than the cho-mo, I was never aware of it.

Atop the pyramid of power, the true shot-callers in prison are the made-guys. The organized crime guys. Never ostentatious, never loud, never bringing attention to themselves. They were not only shown respect and deference to, but they were gentleman themselves. In short, nobody messed with them. Once I was 'vetted' after a few days I was introduced to some of these men and being Italian, I was looked out for. Security is a very precious asset in prison.

But in any group, there are guys who don't follow the rules. Official or otherwise. These are the crazies, the loose cannons, the dangerous ones. These are the guys you need to use vigilance with. Although the word may be out that you're not to be hassled with, really bad things can happen. *You* must be ready. *You* must be on guard. *You* must be prepared. And you can only do that by building a solid, battle-ready physique. When you're locked in a cage with guys fresh off the streets of an urban battleground you know it's not showtime. It's go time, and you better be ready.

Daniel Goleman in his study of emotional intelligence observed "having hope means that one will not give in to overwhelming anxiety, a defeatist attitude or depression in the face of difficult challenges or setbacks." Hope, he writes, is "more than the sunny view that everything will turn out all right;" it is "believing you have the will and the way to accomplish your goals."

In prison those who had hope—hope that they would survive the ordeal, hope that their wives would remain faithful, hope that their children would not turn their backs on them, hope that their appeal would be successful — these were hopes that kept a man moving forward. When you're locked up for years "what doesn't kill me makes me stronger" is more than a phrase. It is a fact. [8]

Eighty million Americans are currently listed on the FBI's Master Criminal Database! This number is incredible! A country of approximately 330,000,000 people has nearly 25 percent of its citizens categorized as criminals! Put another way however, by segregating adults in this number (which includes those under 18) one third of the adult population of the United States are crooks! 9

Although most people can never imagine being incarcerated, 3-5% percent of inmates in the nation's prisons are in fact, innocent! Since most of those charged with a crime "plead out" there is no accurate figures available but there have been unofficial estimates as high as 15-20% wrongfully accused sitting in prison! Over and over, we learn of convicted criminals walking out of prison free men and women due to new evidence, DNA results or recanting witnesses. We hear stories of prosecutorial misconduct such as suborning perjury, forcing confessions and threatening defendants with crushing sentences should they lose at trial that they "plead out" to a lesser sentence, innocence be damned. 10

What is left though, is the opportunity (if we dare call it that) to discover within ourselves, regardless of the circumstances, the ability to not only overcome adversity, anguish, and reversals but to turn those misfortunes into personal empowerment and breathtaking triumph.

Victor Frankl, the Austrian psychiatrist who survived the Holocaust wrote: "When we are no longer able to change a situation, we are challenged to change ourselves." Dr. Frankl was speaking from first-hand experience. He observed his fellow prisoners closely and discovered that those who kept hope, kept thinking that tomorrow would be a better day had (and did have) a better chance of survival. Those who simply gave up and gave in to their circumstances did not.

We all meet with reversals, with frustrations and downfalls. Try as we might to avoid them, they periodically appear in our lives. How do you handle them? Have you ever considered yourself a failure? Have you ever thought "How am I ever get through this one?"

"I am now the most miserable man living. If what I feel were equally distributed to the whole human family, there would not be one cheerful face on the earth. Whether I shall ever be better I cannot tell; I awfully forbode I shall not. To remain as I am is impossible; I must die or be better, it appears to me."

At the time he wrote this, his friends were so concerned about him that they removed razors, knives, and any sharp objects from his room, convinced he would take his own life. No matter how hard he tried, things just would not go his way. It stayed like that for a while for Abraham Lincoln.

What set Lincoln apart however from the 'average guy' was that he did not wallow in self-pity and while away time in idleness. "Fueled by his resilience, conviction and strength of will," writes Doris Kearns Goodwin in her superb book *Team of Rivals,* "Lincoln gradually recovered from his depression."

Based on my life experiences I believe that prison is the most depressing, dismal, saddest place on earth. It is a place where your dreams collide into a brick wall. You live as if in a kind of suspended animation. Almost as in a subterranean tomb where you go through the motions of life while the real world goes on above without you.

I wrote earlier that "if there is a hell on earth, prison comes near to it." What for me *became* hell on earth was losing my wife.

On the outside, in the free world break-ups are never easy. They are brutal, gut-wrenching affairs. It is said that the most difficult experience that can happen to a person is to be rejected. In a 'normal' life you move on, but in a prison cage you become despondent, a feeling of hopelessness descends, and grabs hold of your very soul. Fortunately, through support from family and friends, you eventually emerge from the despair and the gloom. You move forward, however tenuous the steps. God puts a new person in your path and you slowly emerge from the impenetrable darkness. In prison though, there is no "moving on." There is not a smiling face, a gentle voice, not a loving caress or a "somebody new." There is just a loneliness, a mind, and imagination that is firing with mental pictures and images that become more torturous with each passing night.

Losing the woman I adored, whom I never lost my boundless infatuation with, was unbelievably worse than being sentenced to a thirteen-year prison term.

Bishop Desmond Tutu once wrote "Hope is being able to see that there is light despite all of the darkness." I recalled the line from (ironically enough) the movie *The Shawshank Redemption*. The inmate, Red, played by Morgan Freeman opined to either "get busy livin', or get busy dyin." I chose life.

After my legal problems arouse, I began to lose confidence in myself. As the months went by, I experienced reversals that, in my worst nightmares, I could not have envisioned. Adding to these challenges were my health concerns. I was not only despondent over my issues with the government but also weak in every facet of my being.

In hindsight I probably went back to work too soon after coming home from the hospital after the heart attack (although the government raided our offices three months earlier, they did not padlock the doors or force us to close), but I was desperate to protect the investors of WaterMark and trying to get them repaid.

Incredibly, eight of our coworkers, including my son Geoffrey, struggled to right the ship for nearly a year — with no pay! To illustrate the lost vigor and spirit that I once had, there was an incident that took place a few days within returning to the office after my discharge:

I had requested a firm (who I had monetarily assisted over the years) if they might consider working with us in our recovery by offering their particular product to our remaining clients. Along with the company's owner a few other of their principals, including their sales manager, joined us in our conference room. Before we began our meeting, immediately after sitting down actually, this sales manager proceeded to rip me apart, as his voice rose, dripping with vituperation, sarcasm, and condescension. I just sat there. And took it.

After the 'meeting' ended, Geoffrey told me that if it weren't for my inviting them in the first place, he would have thrown the loudmouth out the window. Such is the insidious feeling of shame, embarrassment, and defeat.

I will spare you the countless stories and incidents similar to the one above that I experienced before entering prison. Walking through those forbidding gates at Elkton left me no choice, absolutely no alternative but to "man-up." My life, literally, depended on doing so.

Those who, at one time, were into weight training (but may have stopped for whatever reason) know — or discover — that muscle has memory. Fortunately, so does confidence, self-esteem, and determination. It was in the prison weight room that I discovered how similar life's challenges were to the demands of lifting weights. Perseverance, pain, determination, moving past barriers, setting goals, and achieving those goals—all can be said of life, and weight training as well. It is, in a word: discipline.

During those many years of being locked away I found cryptic, perhaps indiscernible ambiguities, of who I once was and what those discoveries revealed to me. Perhaps you may recognize them in your life. Feeling guilty leads a person to not only expect to be punished but to feel that they deserve to be!

Being remorseful in front of the court is one of the deciding factors the judge uses in handing down a sentence. Personally, I felt horrible for the pain and anguish I had caused to so many, consequently the remorse I felt was genuine. But feeling guilty does no one any good. It can, and often does, render the person paralyzed forevermore. In lockup I saw it. I witnessed guys who at one time were at the top of their chosen profession break, insensible and benumbed never to be the same again. That was a luxury I could not afford.

Branded a liar and a thief I had only myself left to prove anything to. For three years prior to going to prison I read the articles written about me. I absorbed the contempt hurled at me when I ran into someone somehow affected by my actions. I began to despise myself which soon turned to loathing — a feeling that never left me until three years had passed in prison. It was then, a few weeks prior to Christmas in 2014 that I said to myself *"This is enough!"*

That feeling was not a disregard for anyone, but an empowerment that would allow me to "get busy livin'" and strive to accomplish what I knew needed to be done. It isn't practical to expect yourself to be upbeat constantly. Life as we know, is full of changes, challenges, disappointments, and sorrows. It is knowing how to deal with them with wisdom that enables you to overcome them. If a tree has strong roots, deep and anchored firmly, no storm can uproot it.

How do you overcome adversity when it appears? Do you possess mental and emotional toughness? How do you know if you do? There are only two ways, that I know of to endure obstacles and dilemmas and master them: maintain a spiritual connection to God, generally with frequent prayer and possess a high degree of discipline.

When St. Paul began writing letters to the churches he planted at various locations throughout the eastern Mediterranean (many times writing them while he was in prison) he implored those early Christians to always maintain a connection to God. 11

You don't need to "wear your faith on your sleeve" so to speak. Your actions will always speak for you anyway. What matters is your faith and the trust you put in Him that no matter the challenge everything will work out. I have lived by this belief which is what enabled me to survive prison.

Throughout my incarceration I continued to meditate on the following words found in Romans 8:28 "And we know that all things work together for good to those who love God, to those who are called according to His purpose. "Notice that it says "*All things*" not *some* things or *maybe* things can work out. **ALL THINGS**. If there is only one message that you put into practice from this book, I live in hope that it is this one.

Too many people give up on their dreams, their goals, and themselves. Of course, you already know this as well as the obvious reason why — lack of effort. The French Scientist Louis Pasteur, the developer of the process known as pasteurization once observed "Chance favors the prepared mind." Preparation can only come about through effort. You must be willing to do that which is difficult, putting in the effort to set up the outcome you desire. When you move forward toward your goal, set up a first objective. Accomplish that first goal. Make it an easy one. Then go to the next. Realize that one. Go on to the third goal, and so on. When you achieve a goal—no matter how 'easy' or even insignificant, you set your mind up with knowing success. Show gratitude, be exhilarated! You accomplished what you set out to! Don't minimize and if you get negatives from anyone "You only did _____ what's the big deal?" Get that person out of your life. They're dream stealers!

One of the best demonstrations of the results of putting your mind to something, of focusing on achievement and continuing to reach even higher I found to be in the weight room. If you can discipline yourself to train - cardio or weights or a combination of both, you will discipline yourself in many areas of your life!

Weight training is more — much more, actually — demanding on a person than just attempting to bulk up. When lifting weights, the stress placed on the central nervous system (CNS) is in direct proportion to the poundage someone is attempting to lift. The heavier someone trains the greater response from the CNS. As you train, the CNS is processing information and adjusting the corresponding body parts and muscle groups in what really is a miraculous symphony. As you lift, the CNS contracts one muscle while at the same time relaxes another. It balances the body through the move yet keeps a firm grip on the physical movement itself.

It may be hard to believe but a muscle is only as powerful as the signal sent to it from the brain of the person working out. The reason for this is due to the perception the brain has toward danger. If it senses injury to the body, it will withhold explosive power to the muscle. If there is a perception of joint instability due to lack of the proper muscle firing patterns, the CNS will down-regulate power to the muscle.

If you've lifted in the past, you know the feeling of "I don't feel like working out today." If you walk into the gym unenthused or have the feeling of "I'm not that strong," your brain — through the CNS — will adjust to that feeling by down-regulating power to the muscles for that as well. Your mind has enormous power not only on your workout goals but also on your life.

Most people respond positivity through encouragement, visualization, inspiration, and positive self-talk. This is the best reason to associate with people who up-lift you. If you don't have friends like that — make new friends! Your workouts will improve if you maintain an optimistic expectation that they will. Try reading material that motivates you, encourages you, and inspires you. When you have high expectations your actions, as well as workouts, will follow those patterns.

During my career in finance, I constantly searched for ways to improve. I studied new economic theories, became more proficient at reading stock charts and monitored domestic and international events that could — and many times did — affect the U.S. stock markets. I took notes from various financial studies and analyses, and I became adept at listening. Most of all, I listened to my clients. What was important to them, what their goals were, and how we could achieve them. I mention this because when you put your focus on being the best you can be, you do the grunt work. What most people discuss as pointless effort is a natural and normal way of preparation for the one who plans on excelling. Truth be told these people usually don't consider the activity work, but find satisfaction knowing the objective will be attained because of their attention to every detail.

Paying attention to detail is essential. Whether someone is under a 405-pound squat bar or preparing a formal business proposal, they must employ concentration and determination. Both require mentally picturing the end result. Let me state again: When you achieve a goal, you are setting your mind up with knowing success.

But what if you fail?

To most people failure is the greatest of unwanted outcomes. In prison, I repeatedly heard self-depreciating statements: "My life is over. My career is done. Nobody's gonna hire me. I'm broke. By the time I get out of here, I'll be too old." This statement was not exclusive to only one or two people.

I had the "distinction" (dubious I think) of being the guy people could come to when they needed a shoulder to cry on or to get inspired. I got to be known as "St. Gino, the patron saint of lost causes." This was not always meant to be flattering by the way! It was to the point that when trouble was brewing on the compound guys would come find me to mediate. Now remember, it is not wise to get involved in disputes between other inmates – nor did I want to. But most everyone on the compound knew me and hoped I might diffuse a potentially explosive situation, a.k.a. a beating.

Make no mistake in my motives, however. Helping others walk through a problem, deal with sadness, or overcome hopelessness also helped me. The defeatist attitude that was at times found in prison was almost exclusively felt by the white-collar guys. Doctors, lawyers, stockbrokers, politicians, pharmacists as well as pharmaceutical reps, accountants, mortgage brokers, business owners — they were all there. Of course, there was a high degree of truth in the statement "Nobody's gonna hire me." Many of the better paying jobs are more difficult, if not impossible to receive with the noun 'felon' behind your name.

My attitude however, and one that I shared with others was (and is) "When one door closes another opens." Never doubt, not even for a second that we serve a God of not only second chances but twentieth chances, fiftieth chances and eightieth chances!

Failure is an opportunity. If you embrace the hidden message in failure, you can become more emotionally tough and mentally powerful than you can possibly imagine. Pay attention, *pay very close attention* to your failures. You have undoubtedly heard of those who failed, were rejected, met with defeat and (metaphorically) left for dead.

"You ain't goin nowhere, son. You ought to go back to drivin' a truck," said the guy at the Grand Ole Opry when he fired Elvis.

J.K. Rowling was a divorced single mother. She was broke, and like so many of us when you don't know where the next dollar is coming from, depressed. She kept focused on her writing, though, and the *Harry Potter* series she imagined propelled her to become one of the wealthiest women in the world. Rowling once observed "It is impossible to live without failing at something, unless you live so cautiously that you might as well not have lived at all in which case, you fail by default."

Steven Spielberg's dream was to attend USC's School of Cinematic Arts but being rejected twice didn't seem to impede his ability to gross over $9 billion dollars from his movies. He also won three Academy Awards.

It took 5,126 failures over a period of fifteen years before Sir James Dyson created his bagless vacuum cleaner that led to an eventual net worth of $4.5 billion.

Walt Disney was told by his former newspaper editor he lacked imagination.

Oprah Winfrey was fired from her first anchor position at a Baltimore TV Station.

Theodor Geisel's first book was rejected by twenty-seven different publishers. He kept going, and Dr. Seuss went on to sell over 600 million copies of his children's books.

Stephen King's wife retrieved the first book he wrote, *Carrie*, out of the garbage where he dumped it after being rejected thirty times by book publishers. Handing it back to him he kept submitting the manuscript which was eventually published generating his fantastic career.

I could go on and tell you that the first time Jerry Seinfeld stepped on the stage, he froze. The audience booed and jeered him off that stage. Not giving up, he returned the next night and had the audience in stiches. He never looked back.

What about Michael Jordan? He once said "I have missed more than 9,000 shots in my career. I have lost almost 300 games. On twenty-six occasions I have been entrusted to take the game winning shot, and I missed. I have failed over and over again in my life. And that is why I succeed."

Jordan, who was cut from his high school basketball team went on to win six championships and five MVP's and become what many consider the greatest basketball player of all time.

You too have failed. Many times. It happened when you took your first step. When you fell you kept getting up and kept on trying again.

It happened when your parents took the training wheels off of your bike. You may have even cut yourself when you fell, but you still kept climbing back on until you could ride in a straight line.

You struck out playing baseball. You failed tests at school, and you may have failed at love a time or two. You didn't quit, however, you just dug your heels in and kept trying until you succeeded.

No matter how many times you fall, pick yourself up, dust yourself off and keep on running. You are a failure only if you stop trying. When you find yourself face down in the mud put your arms to the side and propel yourself up. A good salesman knows that the "law of averages" never fails. Each time they hear the word "no" they know they are closer to a "yes."

Never give up! Never, ever give up! When you're let go at work, rejoice. God is about to open a new door in your life!

Keep your eyes open, open your ears as well because you'll need all of your senses to hear opportunity creeping up on you.

Stay away, no, disassociate yourself, from negative people and bad influences. You'll never get to the promised land with pessimists holding you back.

So you've made mistakes. What about it? Those mistakes are the means that you use to learn how to do things the right way. Don't be a victim. Forget the sad, forlorn eyed, poor-me look. No one wants to hear sorrows. They have enough of their own.

I witnessed this too many times to count behind the fence. Guys always come in with a shell-shocked look on their face. I understood the heartbreak and fear that a man had walking through the gates. I remembered feeling the same. Six months, eighteen months, three years, ten years, whatever, if it was their first bid it's all relative. Nonetheless to constantly moan to everyone within earshot, especially continuing to do so after a few weeks, became annoying. Offensive, even, to guys who'd been down for decades.

I recall one guy who was having a hard time adjusting. Crying, tears and snot running down his face, he found it hard to hold a conversation. This went on for weeks. I empathized with him, but one day several weeks after he arrived, I happened to be working on my case in the Law Library and there, at the end of a conference table I noticed this same guy sitting there puffy eyed. "How long did you get?" I asked. This was not a question that was usually asked of another inmate as it is a bit intrusive as well as disrespectful. But hearing his whimpering I thought I might be able to extend some encouragement. I had also begun to hear the rumblings from some of the 'long-term' residents on the block about him.

This inmate, about fifty years old or so answered, between sobs "eighteen months." Eighteen months?! I stared at him in disbelief. "You'd be wise to knock this stuff off right now," I said. "There are guys who've been locked up for thirty years here. You've been fussing for weeks all over the yard. You're going to get hurt if you don't knock it off."

For everything and for everyone there is always "a first." The first steps, the first kiss, and, if you're a convicted felon, your first night in jail. It is a traumatizing moment, that first night.

Many years ago, I recall hearing the following: You are either in a major trial right now, you are just coming out of a major trial, or you are about to experience a major trial. I know none of these options sound pleasant but reread the quote from James at the beginning of this section. These trials, mistakes, failures, mess-ups, call them what you will, are a blessing—if you are mentally and emotionally mature enough to see them for what they are. When they happen (*when, not if*) look for the message. You'll find they are filled with meaning and knowledge. Coming from someone who spent the better part of a decade in prison this may sound crazy, but when I counseled the new guys, I said this very thing.

I had many friends on the outside. Hundreds. I was a popular guy. Active in the community. I served on boards of directors, as the president of community and charitable organizations, and was a guest on local and national television. I even had my own radio show. Yea, knew lots of people. Everybody wanted to be around me. The smiles were wide, the hugs big. Success has a way of extending its brilliance to warm those who crowd around you. When it hit the fan — and I say this with complete candor — I could literally count my friends on one hand. But, and this is the blessing, I now know who my *real* friends are. What about you? Who are *your real friends*? Like I said — pay attention to the screw-ups in your life. You will learn more from them than your successes.

"Act as though I am, and I will be." This is a powerful declaration. To put it another way—visualize the end result. "That's crazy!" you say? Not at all. You probably do this more than you realize. Sadly, most people "see" obstacles, problems, and unfulfilled dreams.

Whenever you visualize what you don't want, you likely add strong feeling and emotion to the scenario. When you verbalize statements such as "I'm afraid I won't be able to do it," "I'm in real trouble if I don't pay this," or any number of discouraging remarks, you anchor your subconscious to some sort of loss. Your subconscious does not reason, it acts on the emotion of the order given. "I can't" to the subconscious means "Don't do it." "Maybe" means "You won't." "Why even try?" means "Don't bother, it won't happen anyway." Not having the capacity to discern good outcomes from bad, the subconscious will act on whatever emotions are the strongest.

Think back to our discussion about REM sleep. As you'll recall, REM sleep is the deepest part of sleep where the body recovers and improves itself. It is also the point at which the brain waves are comparable to the real world, as if a person is wide awake!

How many times have you dreamt of something pleasant that seemed so real? Conversely, you'll recall a nightmare so vivid and genuine that you woke up in total fear. Heart pounding, nerves exploding, maybe even panic stricken. This was visualization at its most refined. This was solely a mental experience that took total control of your body and, in that moment, seemed totally real. Remembering such an experience, can you really reject the premise that "where the mind goes, the body follows"?

There are two basic factors that motivate human beings: pain and pleasure. Virtually every person craves pleasure and pursues that feeling often. Although pleasurable experiences are enjoyable, human beings *will do anything* to avoid pain. With this thought in mind is it any surprise that, in order to avoid pain, people put the strongest feelings on unwanted outcomes?

Too many people torture themselves by conjuring negative outcomes. The human brain is wired to avoid injury to the body but why, when given a choice, do most people see bad results instead of the best outcome? Our decisions are made in the part of the brain known as "The Reflexive" brain, located in the right hemisphere. The decisions are often made by our feelings and once we attach our feelings onto risk or fear we greatly magnify the risk or fear. The feeling of negative outcomes is an off-shoot of the fear of uncertainty, but it was that fear that allowed our prehistoric ancestors to survive. They needed food and shelter and having a fear of uncertainty kept our species going. So, you would be safe in saying that thinking of worst-case scenarios is hard-wired into our brain. Fortunately, our Creator gave and gives us free choices. Free choices allow us to choose optimism and positivity. You are free to visualize happy endings and the more you visualize positive outcomes, making it as real as you can the more 'possible' turns into 'probable.' Your imagination is your greatest gift. *No- one* can take it from you. You are free to conjure the best outcomes. The happier you are, the more you feel that the outcome WILL happen as you want. There is more to this story, the path to obtaining and achieving what you desire, and we'll explore that path in a bit.

At different times during your life you've probably been told to "think positive" and "Don't dwell on negatives." You've also been exposed to motivational and self-help books. To get to the place where things flow in an orderly fashion (while allowing for life's challenges and unexpected obstacles) you'll need to learn to discipline your mind, as well as your life, habits, and activities. In order to do this, you must want this. Desperately. Each time you slide back into old habits and thought patterns — and you will — you will need to summon the motive, the basics of the purpose that motivated you to commit to achieve your particular objective or objectives. You will need to not only take charge of what you think but how you think.

Most of us have an inner monologue that runs constantly through our conscious mind. As if on a perpetual audio loop, this inner voice continuously verbalizes our inner feelings, opinions, observations, judgments, and outlook. If you were to examine this internal dialogue, what would you discover about this chatter? You will probably surprise yourself about what you listen to all day, and you'll probably find that your present circumstances align with what you're talking to yourself about.

You see, this is the reason that "pray without ceasing" is not only logical but powerful. Prayer brings God — the power of the universe — into your daily life in a profound and compelling way. Now you may be thinking "If he believes that, why did he end up (or stay for so long) in prison?" If that thought crossed your mind, it's a valid question.

My only answer is *God allows things to happen in our lives*. A simple answer I would give would be that the mistakes I made through my own free will as well as my miseries, my mess-ups, my heartbreaks, and my experiences were lessons I needed to learn. I fully trusted that the years I spent in prison were for a purpose. A purpose greater than "He's a crook who belonged in jail!" I believed then, and I believe in now, the words you can find in Jeremiah 29: 11 "For I know the thoughts I think toward you, says the Lord, thoughts of peace and not of evil, to give you a future and a hope." Whether you are a believer or not, I can attest — through experience — that these words not only hold meaning but are true.

Meditation

In addition to prayer, I found peace of mind in meditation. Over the years in prison, I found ways to leave — if only in my mind — the yard. Music took me away, transcending the gloom and sadness through a piano keyboard. The other means of my whimsical liberation I found in the gym. Meditation, however, brought me into a silence, a freedom, a way to allow God to soak throughout my spirit.

Despite my longing to meditate more frequently, I was usually relegated to the time after lights out to do so. I also stole a few minutes after my cardio workout, following my yoga routine whenever possible, but usually some clown would intentionally intrude with a brainless comment which would bring me back to the present.

When the lights were switched off, I'd sit cross-legged on my bunk, back straight, eyes closed. In order to enter into silence, I would often times need to don earplugs to keep the sounds of lock-up out. Concentrating on my breath, I would soon feel a calmness, a wave of contentment filling me, allowing the day's challenges to drift away. The type of silent sitting I practiced is known as Vipassana meditation.

There are no chants, incense, or incantations — no sound except the softness of your breath. There is no religious dogma attached to Vipassana meditation, just a desire to bring peace and tranquility into your life.

If you are new to meditation, don't give up when a torrent of thoughts intrudes upon your consciousness. Advanced practitioners who have sat in silence for years also experience conscious intrusions. The memories, obligations, pictures, and agitations of your life will suddenly make their presence known. Even music can make its appearance. This is called "Monkey Mind" because like the little monkey who never sits still — reaching for the vine, rolling on the ground, screaming, and just not able to settle down — your mind doesn't like restrictions.

Don't get upset. When this happens simply return your focus on your breath, without annoyance and without anger. Breathe through your nose, concentrate on which nostril is dominant when you breathe (you'll likely be surprised you never took notice of this before) and put your attention to that nostril. Vipassana Meditation was first taught 2,500 years ago by Siddhartha Gautama, Buddha. [12]

There is noise most everywhere on the block or in the yard. Lots of guys talking slick, gossiping, screaming, swearing, and just plain obnoxious. Starting early and lasting past lights out — the reason I'd periodically use earplugs during meditation — the rudeness never ceased to amaze me.

In order to experience some degree of peace and quiet I started my day between 4:30 and 5 a.m. In order to train in the weight room properly, I knew I needed at least seven hours of sleep, so I was usually in my bunk by 10 p.m., often earlier. During my time in prison, I grounded myself in discipline. Everything I did, every work assignment, every task, every responsibility, I did with purpose.

In prison I learned to not live by the good opinion of others. As a former addict — Approval Addict — my habit was to make many, if not most, of my decisions — personal and business — based in pleasing others regardless of the relationship — family members, friends, acquaintances, business associates, and even employees. I tried to please everyone. Going to prison forced me to "get clean."

What I observed, what I experienced, what I heard, and how I was treated throughout all the years of my legal challenges opened my senses to the complete absurdity of striving to be Mr. Congeniality. Most of us, if given a choice want to be respected. We hope to be liked, but if in order to achieve these aspirations our self-worth and our identity become dependent on them, then a period of serious introspection is in order. That self-examination, self-analysis, and soul-searching was achieved completely during my residency in prison.

Over the years, I became aware that my "self" changed, transformed actually, in very profound ways. It wasn't only in my physical condition or my habitual approval fixation but the metamorphose from "intellect-based" to "intuition-based." By this I mean I put more emphasis on how I felt about something. That is not to say I abandoned my power of reason, but to rely on the comfort I felt in my spirit more frequently than I had in the past. It was the "still small voice" Solomon wrote of. Some call it trusting your gut. Others call it intuition. I call it being led by the Holy Spirit.

Although every person's path is different, we can improve the conditions we personally encounter on that path by now and again being mindful of the trials and experiences of another. Sadly, experience is the best teacher, but the wise individual observes and learns from the mistakes and successes of others.

Each of us have heard stories, read about, or even personally know someone who faced overwhelming hardship and not only emerged on the other side but became massively successful. Being successful, by the way, does not always involve having a lot of money. Certainly, money needs to freely revolve around your life experience, but in and of itself, a crinkled piece of green paper or even a steamer trunk full of it doesn't kiss you back and it sure doesn't love you back either.

Success is love. Love is what endures. When you put your head on your pillow at night — or a rolled-up coat in a jail cell — knowing that someone, somewhere loves you, adores you and can't wait to hold you — *that* is true success.

Countless books have been written about motivation, persistence, about becoming better than you've been. Whether you're sitting at dialysis, the unemployment line, the dining room table, or a cabana on the beach, everyone wants to know that through it all they will be better off tomorrow than they are today. How do we achieve that? How does someone arrive at a place and is able to say, "I'm good!" As I see it, it's learning from our mistakes, learning from another person's mistakes, recalling the achievements we've made, learning how others have achieved and finally never, ever giving up — which in the end is not only gratifying but empowering.

It is doing everything impeccably, leaving no regret of "I could've done better." It's working to the very best of your ability. It's about leaving nothing on the table, and nothing left undone. It's about using every accomplishment as a step to build a higher one. It's about taking the garbage, the heartbreaks, the disappointments, the if-onlys, the "I almost….", the insults, and the tears and then, with rock-hard determination, clenched teeth, and a crystal-clear vision, saying "I will!" That, my brothers and sisters, is also success.

So much of life in prison is upside down. You want to be gracious, but kindness is usually taken for weakness. You want to be friendly, but friendliness is usually taken for naivete. You want to be respectful and polite but over-doing respect and being overly polite is usually taken for being an easy mark. The balancing act an individual goes through in prison is one of becoming calloused and suspicious, as well as formidable, while not losing your nature and true character.

Gratitude

Gratitude is a very ambiguous word. You can be thankful for a loving family, and you can be thankful for hitting all the green lights while running late for work. The appreciation is conveyed to both but one is unconditionally more heartfelt. One of life's most profound truth's is that in order to receive even more you need to be grateful for what you already have.

You will recall our discussion on visualization and getting what you don't want. Gratitude has an effect on outcomes. For example, imagine a man that has been living in the same house for seventeen years. That old house has seen better days. The paint is peeling, the furnace is old, and the porch needs fixing. "I hate this dump! Every time I look around something goes wrong. Once I get a new house," he says to no one in particular, "I'll be happy". But let's look more deeply at what is really going on.

He is fed up as well as angry that he has to live in this "dump." But yet at one time our hero was proud of the house he bought and the joy living in it brought him. The house protected him in all kinds of weather. Although it certainly sounds as if he should consider moving, our man should at least be thankful that he has a place of his own and that despite the minor repairs needed, it has appreciated in value.

You see, if you are grateful for what you have now, no matter how seemingly insignificant it may be, you are giving off positive energy. You are actually sending out vibrations of a positive nature and like a magnet you quickly see those vibes come back to you. The longer you dwell on what you don't like, focusing more attention on what you don't want, you can be certain you'll continue to experience even more to not want. The next time you decide to complain about something watch what happens next-something else will "go wrong."

Going back to our homeowner, let's say he does manage to purchase a new home. With thoughts of a negative nature surrounding him he is sure to find a problem with the electrical wiring, a clogged drainpipe, a leak in the roof or a neighbor who not only blasts his music so he can't help but hear it but also a dog who loves to bark constantly. The reason for outcomes like this has to do with the negative radiation surrounding our homeowner. The parameters he has set up in his mind can only attract further disappointments.

It's not enough to declare "I don't want this to happen!" Abstaining from visualizing disappointing scenarios and being grateful for what you already have are a very powerful combination that sets up your corner of the world to experience gratifying outcomes.

As the weeks and months went by after the government raided my office, all could think of is "What if I go to jail?" Soon my fears created "movie scenes" of not only that but what seemed like every scary outcome. "If this happens, then that will happen!"

The more I feared the more real it felt. Have you ever felt anxious, scared really, about something, *hoping* the feeling would disappear and then it happening anyway? What this is about is "reducing importance." Not going to prison was (*very*) important to me, thus I dwelled on an unwanted outcome, mixed it with vivid mental images and a great deal of fear. The more I thought about it, the more I used my imagination, the more important it was to avoid it.

Fortunately, you are not (hopefully) facing prison, however you may encounter confinements of another kind — where to get the money to pay an unexpected medical bill, an overextended checking account or a job loss. In order to reduce importance, take action! Too many people become as paralyzed as the mouse facing the python when confronted by adversities and challenges, deciding to worry instead. Taking steps toward addressing a situation not only gives you some degree of comfort

— a positive, hopeful feeling — but inspires you. It allows you to stop dwelling on a negative outcome and replaces it with a positive one.

Another method of reducing importance is to have insurance — to have a backup plan. This could be as simple as calling the medical billing department to arrange a payment option or calling the bank to work out a plan to stop overdraft fees. In every individual situation, the course of action will be different but there are usually remedies available. Stay calm by knowing an answer will come. An idea will appear. This is what I referred to earlier — choice.

You really do choose your life experiences. Remember who is writing this: someone who spent nearly nine years in a federal prison! I would give anything to believe that I had nothing to do with this. But I can't. The choices I made, who I became business partners with, who I hired, how I managed my business and employees, the decisions *I made* — all of them were my choices. As I've said before, our attitude towards any event determines the reality of our experience.

A person's attitude causes their emotional response. I could choose to look at the years I was incarcerated, for instance, as a total waste made up of only embarrassment, loss of money, abandonment and degradation. Certainly on the superficial level that is true, but while I was lock up, I chose to view my circumstances as a blessing. I certainly did not want to be there, but I found a degree of peace and a higher degree of wisdom knowing who truly cared for me, who truly loved me. I took the time to look inward, to not only regain my health but to get into the best physical shape of my life. Being incarcerated allowed me to reflect back on my life – all the way back to my childhood. I was able to recall too many instances as I was growing up where I strove for everybody's good opinion of me. It became clear where all of that approval addiction began to take shape. In prison I took charge of what I was able to still control of my life. I decided to write books, to become certified as a fitness trainer, and to create and write courses of study. I was able to explore deeply my Christian faith and my relationship with God.

Whatever challenges you are facing, or may face in the future, keep the following in mind: Don't fight obstacles; overcome them by reducing the importance you place on them. This is accomplished by taking actions to solve the problem and, when possible, having a fail-safe option, a secondary back-up plan. Become accustomed to listening to — and being led by — the "still small voice," the Creator of the Universe imbued in each of us.

There is a quote that you may have heard in the past: "If you want something bad enough, you'll get it." I agree with that statement.

Kind of.

No one wanted to avoid prison more than I did. I'm sure most inmates felt just as I did, but not more. I filed appeals, strong ones that carried valid arguments. I visualized my release, what I would do when I got home. Yet the appeals were not successful. How can this be? When you want something so badly, when you want something not to come about why does it? Of course, placing so much importance skews the attainment, as I explained above. But, in the final summary it is this: *"If it is God's will or he allows it'.* Deuteronomy 11:26-28 NKJV   James 4:15 NKJV

While I was firmly ensconced in my government's cloister, I studied. And read. Voraciously. I took notes, I contemplated on what I read. I tried to reconstruct the messages I'd received from my reading to fit my own understandings, usually unsuccessful, but always illuminating. I came to discover, then believe, and eventually, after countless hours of concentrating on what I interpreted, came to know, that God's influence over our lives is undeniable. Whether you are a believer or not, whether you accept Him or not, whether you call Him "The Universal Intelligence," or any of the other countless names He can be known by — His prominence is omnipotent in every human life.

I don't write this as an attempt to evangelize anyone. That is a journey that is, at the end, decided by an individual. It does however explain the unfathomable answers and knowledge given to us at times. Have you ever made a logical decision? You worked out the analytics, and past experiences confirmed (in your mind anyway) that you were taking the correct action towards something. Then you proceed.

Suddenly you feel you could have gone about things differently. Suddenly you feel you made the wrong decision. The problem is now you are too late to change it. This scenario happens all too often.

Usually, prior to making a decision, people feel an uneasiness, a discomfort. Most people put this feeling off to a case of the nerves so they go forward (or don't do) with the plan or idea only to powerfully discover later that the still small voice, the gut feeling should have been followed.

Sound familiar?

The problem (if we can use that word) with making decisions *exclusively* by logic is that the mind has a variety of factors weighing on it — reasoning, "common sense," outside stress, and anxieties just to name a few. The dilemma we face is in knowing which hunch is the right one. Is it the analytical, logical conclusions or is it the inner voice?

I have come to find the best course of action is to take the time to consider the next step. This should not be a one sit-down assignment but an opportunity to not only gather your logical thoughts but to discern what you are inwardly feeling. I use what I call, the "Forty-eight-hour window."

Trying to formulate a solid, well-thought-out decision as well as an effective strategy or plan usually cannot be accomplished in a matter of minutes. Usually not even in a few hours. A period of forty-eight hours allows you time to sort out your personal opinions and perceptions, the pros and cons. It allows you the opportunity to listen to that still small voice. Significantly though it allows you to sleep on it for two nights.

Using forty-eight hours is generally enough time to put your mind at ease in order to avoid any pressure or feeling rushed. The substantial advantage taking this amount of time offers is the ability to logically sort through choices, as well as allowing your emotions and feelings to acknowledge your comfort level.

Of course, there are situations when an instant decision needs to be made and at that moment, we need to rely on whatever data is available to us at that moment. If at all possible, however, taking the time to think and weigh your options is superior to anything else. Through sincere and intense reflection, as well as living with the consequences of ignoring them, I *know* these words to be true.

As you've read this last chapter, you may wonder why I chose to be philosophical in a book ostensibly devoted to health and strength. And to some extent prison life as well. ***It is about building a foundation.***

You will discover a parallel between working out—whether it's cardio training, weightlifting, or a combination of both — and living a life on purpose, being inspired and with enthusiasm. It is about commitment and determination—both crucial components in living and lifting.

You see, if you commit to being a new person — regardless of your age — in the weight room, the same attitude can't help but cross over to your every-day life. There is an attitude that you learn working out that imparts a feeling of confidence knowing you were "able to lift that" which will emphatically and assuredly become part of you.

You are *NEVER too old* to start or start over working to get healthy, to get strong and to take charge of *your life*. Age is nothing more than a number.

If you are just beginning to weight or cardio train, keep two very important points in mind: *easy does it* and accept that it will take time to see results. Although you will notice a difference in your musculature within two months, it will take more time to see massive results. Your diet will need to aid your training. Working hard and eating bad is not only counterproductive but, to put it bluntly, it's stupid. Your supplements will need to be tailored to your workout goal as well as your lifestyle.

Persistence is the key. Expect "off days." Be open to the fact that they will happen, that you just can't do what you were able to do the last time you worked that body part. The good news however is there will also be days when everything is "on" and you have a tremendous workout! They happen too! Through it all be persistent. Good days, bad days, consistency makes a big difference.

Whether it's the board room or the mail room, bring the determination and discipline you learn in the weight room to every aspect in your life.

Build on each small success, each additional increase of weight on the bar, and every extra minute on the elliptical. You won't be able to hold yourself back from becoming — and being — an achiever. Pledge yourself to being the very best you can be and watch the results in *every area of your life!* They will truly amaze and astound you.

Part II

BODY WEIGHT WORKOUT

Every day bite off more than you can chew,

and chew it!

-Anonymous

You're probably familiar with the phrase "doin' hard time." If you are sitting in your cubicle or cell all evening staring at the walls — you're doin' hard time. If you're finished with work, then run to your rack and lay around the rest of the day — you're doin' hard time.

Behind bars if you don't keep busy, you'll regress. You can develop severe psychological problems with depression as a constant disorder. Going 'stir crazy' is usually referred to spending an extended amount of time in solitary, but I've seen guys who just couldn't cope with being in prison go stir crazy too. When you're doing time, you must adjust quickly, and it becomes more manageable if you find an outlet. It could be gambling—not condoned per prison regulations but the staff usually looked the other way. It could be music—the guitar as a popular instrument. However, it was the weight pile that generally attracted the most attention.

Although most guys wandered to the cardio room, finding those really committed to working out there was rare. Weights were more structured and as I wrote earlier, guys were either not allowed in or were shown the door if they weren't showing heart.

Another issue *I found myself* confronting was selfishness with the weights and machines. Every now and then some jag-off would decide that they would place all the dumbbells in front of them—*and keep them there!* In order to avoid problems in lock-up you *must* share. Another goofball decided that he would "circuit-train" with the various apparatuses and weights. In order to be respectful of each other, we would train one body-part per day. Mondays were my shoulder day for instance. Tuesdays were legs. This guy decided he would just use whatever he wanted, when he wanted without regard for anyone. When, after about ten days *I* finally had enough (and this after politely reminding him a few times), that we didn't do this kind of stuff, I confronted him in a not-too-pleasant-way. The other guys there backed me up and we threw him out.

Finding the time to work out could become difficult at times. There were counts, lockdowns, recalls and any sort of emergency found on a prison compound that could delay or cancel your time to lift or train. There are times when the yard is closed for days. I recall a significant dust-up at Schuylkill that caused the cardio room and weight pit to be off limits for twelve weeks!

As annoying as these lockouts could be, (although that twelve weeks was not to be the longest, as it turned out) and the workout areas being a frequent target of retribution, the hardened but committed person could always find a way to get it done!

Body weight training can be done in a cell, a family room, or a hotel room. If someone is determined to be in the best physical shape possible or maintain their strength, body weight resistance is one of the best ways to augment that goal. Body weight can be used as a stand-alone workout or in conjunction with cardio and weight training.

One of the real advantages of body weight training is the safety of the movement. In short this means that the individual's body structure will determine the movement of that individual's muscles and joints. Since there are no 'free' weights to consider, a natural range of motion occurs and with less of a strain on joints, tendons and ligaments.

Most body weight exercises are considered compound exercises meaning that several muscle groups are worked simultaneously. Great physiques aren't constructed in a day, but it's in your hands to take the first step today. Now. Soon you'll like what you see.

BURPEES

When I was a kid, we used to call these 'squat thrusts' but whatever name you use you're probably familiar with this movement. Burpees are a compound exercise and as such causes an increase in testosterone due to the multiple muscle groups called into action. Burpees are an interval training method and has a very beneficial aerobic (increase of oxygen) effect on the body.

EXECUTION

Step 1   Drop down to a squatting position onto your hands,
                knees below the torso

Step 2   Quickly kick both legs back into push up position

Step 3   Quickly bring the knees back to the torso, into a
                squatting position

Step 4   Stand

Step 5   Repeat

Although there are a variety of optional movements with burpees (in step 2, some do one pushup before bringing the knees back to the torso for instance and others may had a jump at the end when they are standing) the original four-step burpee accomplishes the goal of working the core, building endurance, and increasing muscle mass. Use a thin, cushioned mat for landing your hands. Doing so will prevent pressure and strain on your wrists.

PULL UPS

One of the most performed body weight movements in prison is the pull up. Whenever there is an exposed water pipe, support beam or stabilizer bar over a bunk a con will be found banging out multiple sets of these. Performing pull-ups during a lockdown for an extended restriction of rec was an effective way to keep the back and shoulders in tone by using what was available on the block. The pull-up bar in the cardio room was, of course, the best place to do pull-ups but when events dictate otherwise, you use what you can.

Pull-ups will build huge shoulders and a dramatic V-tapered back. Pull-ups are executed with the palms facing away from you. Starting at the bottom, arms fully extended, pull your body up until your chin is over the bar. Lower yourself back to the starting position and repeat.

Chin ups are different only in the placement of your palms which in this exercise are facing you. In addition to working the shoulders and upper back your biceps will also come into play. For a look that projects strength in someone's rear-view mirror or walking up a flight of stairs, pull-ups and chin-ups will nail it.

DIPS

Another go-to exercise behind the fence is called the parallel bar dip.

This movement entails grasping the handles of a 'dip bar' and lifting your body by straightening your arms. Taking a deep breath into your core, bend your elbows and lower your body until your upper arms are parallel to the floor. After a slight pause at the bottom, raise yourself by straightening the arms once again.

Guys on the inside perform dips off the edge of the rack, between washers or dryers, off of two chairs or between two stacks of books. A dip bar is best for this movement, but any stable base will suffice. In a traditional dip work out your feet are suspended in mid-air, never touching a solid object (such as a footstool or crossbar) until the set is complete. However, a beginner should have their feet on the ground while performing this exercise.

Dips will directly affect the chest and shoulders as well as the triceps. Leaning forward will focus on the chest and front deltoids. Performing dips while keeping the back straight will focus on the triceps. 15

JUMPING JACKS

Performing jumping jacks takes up a minimal amount of space making them an acceptable alternative to cardio room access – an important advantage during a prison lockdown.

SQUATS

Normally thought of as a squat rack exercise — walk into the rack, position yourself under the bar and begin to work. But when traditional weighted squats are not possible body weight squats are a decent stand-in.

Body weight squats are simple to perform — hands on hips, legs shoulder-width apart. Squat down until your quads are parallel to the floor. No lower! There are a number of places that talk about the 'benefits' of going below parallel both in body weight and traditional squats but I'm not sure what benefit you receive by putting stress on your knees! This is a controlled movement so be mindful as you perform them. 'Bouncing' off your knees is dangerous and not very intelligent.

Another variation that not only develops leg strength but also balance entails placing the hands, fingers interlocked behind the head. This squat is known as, appropriately, the prisoner squat.

CALVES

A man's calves say a lot about the man. Most guys walk around in Bermudas oblivious to the message their legs, specifically their calves (Bermudas usually hide the quads) send. If their calves are smooth, round and undefined you can be assured that they are not lifting, (regardless of a big chest or large biceps) properly.

Like the squat there are specific exercises that focus on the calves when using weights, however when weights aren't available simply raise your body onto your toes. If you're new to this, place your hands on the wall to stabilize yourself until your CNS becomes accustomed to the move. This should happen fairly quickly.

LUNGES

Although lunges are routinely done with weights — dumbbells, kettlebells or barbell — they are also an excellent body weight exercise. Actually, if you've never performed lunges it would be best to begin with your body weight.

The body needs to feel secure when performing something new so if you've not done lunges before have a bench or something sturdy accessible to get "the feel" of doing them. This is akin to gaining your form when your weight training with an empty bar.

Lunges can, and do, build massive quads but if done incorrectly can cause injury to the knees and adductor muscles (located in the interior of the thighs) as well as cause imbalance. The hip flexors come into play as well. Keep in mind that you are doing this movement, or any training movement for that matter, for you. You are not competing against anyone!

Stand with your feet shoulder-width apart. Bring one leg forward, bending at your knee. Return to the starting position and bring the other leg forward. Do not lean forward or look down as this may cause you to fall forward. Keep your eyes forward, head and back straight as you observe this move with your peripheral vision. Do not bend lower than ninety degrees and do not allow your bent-knee to pass further than your opposite toe.

ABDOMINALS

With the exception of a fully toned and jacked body, nothing seems to attract attention like an abdominal six-pack. Ask 98 percent of the guys in the joint (the other 2 percent? Well, you know) why they workout and the majority say because of women, and nothing seems to attract a woman more than a cut-up midsection on a shirtless guy!

Behind the fence every con knows that a strong deterrent to being hassled, picked on or in some way abused includes a continuous punishment to their body in the workout room. Part of that punishment includes serious ab work.

This is another body weight routine that doesn't require a lot of space for anything more than a towel to lay on. Abdominal movements are considered "core" work and the importance of a strong core cannot be overstated. Additional core exercises are discussed later, but for now let's talk about a few exercises that will increase strength the jailhouse way.

CRUNCHES

Crunches are foundational movements that turns soft muscle into a formidable chassis of body armor. To perform them interlock your fingers behind your head and use them *as a support* as you raise your torso. The idea here is to prevent neck strain while being careful not to "pull" yourself up. Neck injuries are serious so the goal here is to cradle your head during the move. Aiding the movement by pulling the head up is counterproductive as well, due to the shift of focus from the abdominal to the neck.

When performing crunches some like to cross their feet after raising them off the floor while others plant their feet flat on the floor.

You'll be aware of the effectiveness of your work by the tension you'll experience on the abs.

LEG RAISES

The lower abs as well as the hip flexors become the target of leg raises. These are performed by lying flat on the floor, hands under your butt, legs raised six inches off the floor. Count to ten and lower your feet to the starting position.

FLUTTER KICKS

This variation of leg raises will test your commitment to achieving abdominal strength. The idea here is to kick your feet up and down for a ten count and repeat for reps.

SCISSORS

Another style of leg raises, this time by crisscrossing the legs, six inches off the floor.

Abdominal work is about as grueling a workout possible when beginning a total body makeover. The same can be said after a long layoff. When you've completed them however there is a strong sense of accomplishment- as well there should be.

It takes real effort, as well as dedication, to perform ab work but leg-above-the-floor raises especially.

Start out with three separate sets of some type of leg raise five to eight raises per set. Work yourself up to fifteen raises per set, three times per week. For added strength and endurance place your hands behind your head and do not bend your knees. You'll feel the burn at the focal points: lower abs and hip flexors. Upper quads as well.

To get jacked you must put aside the old mindset you once had —"these hurt" — and replace it with the vision of a rock-solid midsection.

REVERSE CRUNCH

This movement focuses on the lower abs-the bottom portion of your Rectus Abdominis. It also trains the Transverse Abdominis which is the innermost abdominal muscle (the muscle inside). Lie on your back hands behind the head elbows wide and pressing the lower back into the floor and raise your legs off the floor, knees bent at a ninety-degree angle toward your chest. Do not use momentum here and for a real midsection burn try lowering the feet to just above the floor after every rep, shoulders lifted off the floor slightly and legs straight (knees unbent)

HANGING KNEE RAISES

The old-school routine of moves that will do the job on abdominals are hanging knee raises. Grasp a pull-up bar, legs strait. Bring the knees up parallel to the floor as the abs begin contracting. Return to the start position and repeat. This exercise can also be performed on a knee raise platform using the same technique but for a con sitting in a cell during a lockdown or a guy working out at home the edge of a bed, a sturdy bench or a heavy chair can get the work in as well.

PUSH UPS

Let's keep it real and concede that there are those whose budgets won't allow for quality but expensive fitness machines, gym memberships, or personal trainers. Some people arising out of this dilemma become frustrated, so much so, that they think "Why bother?"

If this sounds familiar allow me to assure you that you don't need money to get into amazing shape. What you *do need* is the desire to do so. Combined with commitment, dedication, persistence, and visualization your desire ***will become fact***!

When we were on lockdown — a much too frequent occurrence as I've repeatedly pointed out throughout these pages — those of us who took our workouts seriously could find a way to get the work in.

Whether you're a street soldier or a desk jockey you can achieve the broad-shouldered, lean and hungry look that screams of respect. One of the single most effective, perhaps the ***most*** effective all-around exercise is the push-up.

The push-up is not only a strength exercise but an endurance one as well. The chest, shoulders, and triceps are the primary beneficiaries of this move, but push-ups require the kind of cardiovascular endurance that is beneficial to optimal heart health.

According to a recent study in the *Journal of the American Medical Association's Network Open* middle-aged men who are able to complete forty or more consecutive push-ups have a significantly lower risk of heart problems.

Push-ups force you to employ core stabilization unlike a bench press where your body rests on a bench. Form is important as your spine must be in a straight line, hips neither too high nor too low. The neck should be relaxed yet aligned with the spine. If you are experienced at this move, great! However those just starting:

Position your arms under your shoulders or slightly beyond, whichever is more comfortable. Your feet can be wide apart which can help ease into the movement or if you wish, knees on the floor, but I advise starting with correct form at the outset – feet together.

Keep your palms flat on the ground, fingers splayed out which will distribute your weight evenly. Get a full range of motion, elbows out at about a forty-five-degree angle. You can start in an elevated position meaning your hands are on a bench (or any higher, stable object which will make the move easier) but again my advice is to start off in the correct stance, even if you are able to perform only one or two reps.

You will need to know what your maximum consecutive push-ups are before you are totally exhausted or out of breath. If it turns out to be one or two, then it's one or two. Chances are there are more.

In the first week do 70 percent of your max reps, so if that number is five reps, you perform three sets of three reps, rest sixty seconds between sets if you must — but thirty seconds would be better.

The second week should see an increase to three sets of four reps (90 percent). Your goal should be ten reps per set and with persistence and commitment you should achieve this within a few weeks.

If you are already performing ten reps, use the same formula: 70 percent the first week and 90 percent the second, three sets three times per week. Continue to increase your reps. With dedication you will reach your own personal push-up goal.

Once you achieve your objective you may want to incorporate one or two of the following push-up variations:

WIDE SHOULDER PUSH UPS

Placing your hands a bit wider than above will develop rock-hard pectorals and delts the size of coconuts.

DIAMOND PUSH UPS

Place your thumb and forefingers of both hands below your chest forming a diamond shape. This variation targets the inner chest as well as the triceps muscles.

KNUCKLE PUSH UPS

Some of the hardcore cons performed this push-up variation which can result in a slab of steel being thrown in a fight. The muscles in the forearms are brought into play here, but what makes this type of push-up attractive to guys in the yard is the toughening of the skin over the knuckles. Do enough of these and calluses begin to form over the knuckle as well. Some guys would perform these on concrete. I even heard of others doing them *on gravel*! Not to get graphic here but when the knuckle has thick calluses the risk of injury to the knuckle is diminished. In a fight, teeth and nasal bones will cut into the knuckle and really tear them up. As you can imagine the resulting punch got ugly as well as messy.

PLYO PUSH UPS

Plyo push-ups is short for plyometric. For a guy looking for ballistic strength, plyo push-ups are the movement of choice. This move entails explosively pushing yourself up so that the hands and chest are airborne. Done on the floor for maximum training, you can also use a very sturdy bench which reduces resistance up to 40 percent of your body weight.

Start with arms shoulder-width apart (no wider as the downward movement caused by the move could cause shoulder injury). As soon as your chest touches the floor (or bench) explosively launch yourself up again, catching yourself downward as your chest again touches the floor or bench. Repeat for reps.

Using your body as a workout tool is a great way to mix up your workout routine as well as to enhance your overall fitness. The advantage of body-weight training is it can be performed anywhere. In lock-up it kept me conditioned and helped to minimize downtime from the weight pile. In the absence of free weights there is no doubt that just performing form-perfect, high rep sets of pull-ups, dips and push-ups will create and maintain an imposing physique.

In order to continue to make progress however, the body requires variation and relying on body weight only, will cause your gains to stall.

Our muscles need to be challenged and in order to encourage muscular growth, free weights need to be engaged. A well thought out weight training routine involves training the whole body not just the "showy" stuff.

Years ago, "No pain, No gain" was a popular saying. Although soreness is not a pleasant feeling, it does allow us to know the muscles targeted and that the exercise is working.

Pain is one thing, but if working through an exercise is painful — sharp, severe or excruciating —back off. When I visited a health club now and again over the years, I would become infuriated to observe a new member getting "the treatment" by a "trainer." Beat up is more like it. Using too heavy of weights, too many sets, clearly not able to handle the workout. After a workout like that, especially if the person never picked up a weight or trained on a cardio machine before who would be surprised that they never showed up again? Who could blame them? [16]

In order to begin building a solid foundation of muscle or to jump-start after a long layoff, a routine of basic exercises will help you develop physical endurance and a mental mindset that shouts "anything is possible!"

That affirmation will carry over into other facets of your life. Be open to it. Embrace it. Count on it.

WEIGHTLIFTING

IT NEVER GETS EASIER. YOU JUST KEEP GETTING STRONGER

-Unknown

Have you ever noticed that when you are successful in overcoming a difficulty you feel really good about it? Actually, you feel fantastic! Empowered. Inspired even, to do more?

When you go through a genuinely demanding — even painful — experience, everything else seems easy? Or at least, easier? Weightlifting is like that.

Throughout these pages I've related how inmates look at and judge the other cons they come into contact with. They also judge by their work ethic, the weight-pit work ethic. They observe. Not much goes on in prison that's not noticed by every guy. Not only in the yard or on the block. The whole compound. Known as *inmate.com* everyone seems to know what's going on, going down, or about to.

Through inmate.com I discovered that my reputation around the compound was in general, one of respect. That's not to say that everybody loved me. Or even liked me. I can assure you that WAS NOT the case. The great thing (for me anyway) is I had learned to not live by anyone's good opinion of me any longer.

Although most, if not all, human beings are wired to be liked, being respected is, in the end, much more important. In prison it's not only important. It can keep you in one piece.

My work ethic — in the cardio room, at the weight pile, at my job, my Christian faith and involvement with the church — all spoke of who I was. And am. I am not writing this to tell you how great I am or to impress you, but to impress upon you to be all in. All it takes is discipline and among the things I learned in prison, first among them was personal discipline.

The buzz around the compound was that I worked out hard. Really hard. Eventually I was moving big numbers. "You're noticed around the yard" one guy who I hardly knew said to me one day. Let's call it for what it is — they saw the 'old guy' breakin' his butt and getting lean as well as strong. Although I was in my sixties, I felt like I was thirty and thought (still do) like a seventeen year old. My energy level had always been high, but I brought even that up a few notches. Age was and is a state of mind. A number on your prison ID or Driver's License. The only numbers I cared about were the ones on the plates or the dumbbells.

When I entered prison, I was out of shape, weak, heartbroken and a few years on from a massive heart attack. I made a commitment to myself to not only man up but to shape up. I took the failures I made, the hurts I endured and the-yet-unfulfilled goals I had and put them into the iron. The pig iron. If I could conquer my dilapidated and neglected body,

129

I reasoned, I can prove to myself that, with God's help, I could do anything.

Here is how it began: When I walked into the weight room at Schuylkill the day I arrived at the Camp, my first thought was "I can't wait to get started." The next day I did. Over the next ten days or so I just wanted to get reacquainted with the weights, the bars and the dumbbells. There were no fancy machines, no modern equipment at all. Just like a hard-core gym there was a squat rack, a couple of (beat-up) benches, a leg press, a leg extension, dumbbells and a whole lot of free weights.

Everything seemed heavy, even the bar. Form, technique and retraining my central nervous system was going to take time and in the slammer, time is what you have.

I needed to begin training not only smart but focused. Every body part had to be worked but that individualized attention to the separate muscle group would have to wait for a bit.

Determined to "do it right" I recognized that I would have to train my whole body and do so three times a week to start. I followed a plan that would help me train in cycles—a beginner's cycle through advanced. Here-with is the workout program that allowed me to make continuous progress at the weight-pile and, I believe, will do so for you.

As an aside – bring a workout *sheet* with you with the various exercises you will be doing that day. Have everything prewritten on that sheet. After you've finished working a set, write down how many reps you completed. Have a spiral notebook of some sort at home and transcribe that day's workout onto it. This will be your permanent record which you will refer back to time and again.

Before you begin your sets, be sure to warm-up. Stretching and moving light weights prior to your actual routine will minimize the chance for muscle tears and worse – injury. Take at least 10 – 15 minutes to do so.

The following workout, which I began two weeks after I arrived at Schuylkill, is designed to be performed three times per week with at least one day of rest between.

CYCLE 1

MUSCLE GROUP	EXERCISE	SETS	REPS	REST
SHOULDERS	BARBELL SHOULDER PRESS	3	10	2-3 MIN
LEGS	SQUAT	3	10	2-3 MIN
TRICEPS	KICK BACKS	3	10	2-3 MIN
CHEST	BARBELL BENCH PRESS	3	10	2-3 MIN
BACK	BENTOVER BARBELL ROW	3	10	2-3 MIN
BICEPS	BARBELL CURL*	3	10	2-3 MIN
CALVES	STANDING CALF RAISE	3	10	2-3 MIN

*AN EZ CURL BAR CAN ALSO BE USED

This cycle is designed to be worked for weeks one and two. Do not use heavy weights at this time. The standard barbell-known as an Olympic Bar – weighs forty-five pounds. You are not looking to hit your max weight yet. Your goal now is to allow your body and CNS to absorb the feeling of weight training.

In order to grow, muscles need to be challenged. With two weeks of training – which allowed those muscles to learn how to contract in unison – you've learned how to lift, pull and work your legs. You may be a bit sore (CONGRATULATIONS!) which confirms you're working hard! You have been consistent with your workouts and you're not allowing excuses – or others - to impede your progress. That's awesome!

In the second cycle you will be moving to a two-day training schedule. This means you will work your entire body between two separate work outs. You will be working out four days a week now, working each muscle group twice a week. Commitment, dedication and persistence. You need to embrace all these from now on.

CYCLE 2
Workout 1

MUSCLE GROUP	EXERCISE	SETS	REPS	REST
SHOULDERS	BARBELL SHOULDER PRESS	3	8	2-3 MIN
	DUMBBELL LATERAL RAISE	3	10	2-3 MIN
BACK	BARBELL BENTOVER ROW	3	10	2-3 MIN
	1-ARM DUMBELL ROW	3	10	2-3 MIN
CHEST	BENCH PRESS	3	8	2-3 MIN
	INCLINE DUMBELL FLYE	3	10	2-3 MIN
TRAPEZIUS	BARBELL SHRUG	3	10	2-3 MIN

As you can see this workout is a bit more intense than Cycle 1. You should be able to add a bit more weight to the bar, however as

132

you've heard me say - easy does it. Do not sacrifice form and technique by adding too much weight. For instance, you'll notice guys at the gym cutting their bench press high. Instead of bringing the weight down to their chest, lightly touching the chest, they'll come down several inches from the top and go back up. Avoid cheating. Workout the right way. Knowing when to progress up in weight is important. Known as the 2-for-2 Rule, this states that if you can successfully complete two or more reps in the last set in two consecutive workouts for any given exercise, you can increase the weight. [17]

Workout 1 should be done several days apart, say Monday and Thursday. Workout 2 then could be done Tuesday and Friday allowing Wednesday, Saturday and Sunday for rest and recovery.

Note also that instead of performing ten reps on the Shoulder Press and the Bench Press, eight reps are given. This will allow for the slight increase in weight you will have loaded on the bar.

CYCLE 2

Workout 2

MUSCLE GROUP	EXERCISE	SETS	REPS	REST
LEGS	SQUAT	3	8	2-3 MIN
	LEG EXTENSIONS	3	10	2-3 MIN
BICEPS	BARBELL/EZ BAR CURL	3	10	2-3 MIN
	INCLINE DUMBBELL CURL	3	10	2-3 MIN
TRICEPS	CLOSE-GRIP BENCH PRESS	3	8	2-3 MIN
	KICK BACKS	3	10	2-3 MIN
CALVES	STANDING CALF RAISE	3	15	1-2 MIN
	SEATED CALF RAISE	3	15	1-2 MIN

As you can see the moves are becoming more varied. You will want to record your workouts and results as I wrote earlier. This will allow you to track your successes as well as challenges. Remember – these notes are for you so you can be very explicit. The more information you give yourself the easier it is to zero-in on sticking points.

When I was first introduced to this eight-week training course years ago, I was amazed with the inclusiveness of the workouts in relationship to muscle groups, sets, and reps. In addition, as you start out, the rest between sets allows the CNS to recover as well as the ability for you to complete more reps with consistently heavier weights.

By the third cycle your CNS and muscles are becoming accustomed to weight training. You should be very proud of yourself.

You've been persistent when it is very easy to say, "this is work" and blow off a workout.

As I wrote earlier, when a guy wanted to train in prison, they just didn't go to the iron-pit and grab a bar. They had to be invited by a guy already training. This took place quickly for me fortunately. If someone showed proper desire, they could come back.

However, that said, there were plenty of guys who started out with enthusiasm but within weeks (usually within three) they didn't come back. For me personally when I was asked if I could train someone, they had to show heart, lots and lots of heart.

As I referred to previously, lifting was MY time. My release from prison. If the person didn't show passion and intensity, I sent them on their way. That didn't happen often but when it did, I cut them loose quickly.

Weight training involves exercises to maximize muscle growth and to do so using the most effective method. Each workout from this point forward will focus on what is known as push-pull-legs. Basically, this means one day is devoted to the pushing muscles—shoulders, chest, and triceps. The pull day—back, triceps, biceps, and forearms. And the leg day—legs and calves.

These workouts are now spread out over a three-day period, but each day devoted to pushing, pulling, and legs.

Give yourself a day off between each workout for rest and recovery.

CYCLE 3

Workout 1

MUSCLE GROUP	EXERCISE	SETS	REPS	REST
CHEST	BENCH PRESS	3	8	2-3 MIN
	INCLINE D/B BENCH PRESS	3	6	2-3 MIN
	INCLINE D/B FLYE	3	10	2-3 MIN
TRICEPS	CLOSE GRIP BENCH PRESS	3	8	2-3 MIN
	D/B OVERHEAD TRICEPS EXTENSION	3	10	2-3 MIN
	KICK BACKS	3	10	2-3 MIN
SHOULDERS	BARBELL SHOULDER PRESS	3	10-12	1-2 MIN
	D/B LATERAL RAISE	3	10-12	1-2 MIN

CYCLE 3

Workout 2

MUSCLE GROUP	EXERCISE	SETS	REPS	REST
LEGS	SQUAT	3	8	2-3 MIN
	LEG PRESS	3	10	2-3 MIN
	LEG EXTENSIONS	3	10	2-3 MIN
	LYING LEG CURL	3	10-12	2-3 MIN
CALVES	STANDING CALF RAISE	3	15-20	1-2 MIN
	SEATED CALF RAISE	3	15-20	1-2 MIN

CYCLE 3

Workout 3

MUSCLE GROUP	EXERCISE	SETS	REPS	REST
BICEPS	BARBELL/EZ BAR CURLS	3	8	2-3 MIN
	INCLINE D/B CURL	3	6	2-3 MIN
	PREACHER CURLS	3	10	2-3 MIN
BACK	BARBELL BENTOVER ROWS	3	8	2-3 MIN
	1-ARM BARBELL ROW	3	10	2-3 MIN
TRAPS	BARBELL SHRUG	3	10	2-3 MIN
FOREARMS	WRIST CURL	3	10-12	1-2 MIN

You have, by this point in your training, become comfortable moving weights. You've acquired a 'feel' for weight training as well as a sense of satisfaction in doing so. You've been persistent and focused on your goal of taking your body from flab to fabulous.

When I was presented with this workout routine it helped me tremendously. From what I understand this particular workout was helpful to a lot of guys over the years. Wherever it came from, it worked! That said I would encourage you to begin reading beyond this book. Fitness websites are going to be really helpful and magazines – if available - are reasonably priced, packed with workout suggestions and routines and will continue to motivate you.

All of the workouts I presented are geared to the weights and limited equipment we had available in prison. On the street, in most gyms, there are cable machines, lat pulldown machines, smith machines and so much more to help you grow faster, and stronger.

We made do with that we had, and we also devised exercises and moves to supplant our lack of machines. Necessity, they say, is the mother of invention, and I don't believe there are more inventive guys than a bunch of prisoners.

The following workouts are geared to take advantage of the gains you've made over the last six weeks. Stay strict. Good form, proper, healthful diet and good quality supplements. By this point you should be inhaling protein. Meat and premium whey protein should be part of your daily intake - 1 gram of protein per pound of body weight.

Cycle 4 is broken down to four days per week. You will now be working your entire body during these four days. Actually, the only thing missing in these workouts are abdominal training. I trained abs during my cardio workout for a few reasons. As I've written, in lockup there are always recalls back to the block, the training areas being closed because of some trouble on the compound causing daily "normal" schedules to go upside down. Ab work can be done in small spaces like a cell or cube making it hard to make excuses for not doing them. The other reasons I liked doing ab work—and I devoted about thirty minutes on abs six days a week during my cardio workout—was the time constraint at the weight pile. I was always mindful of the next group of guys waiting to workout.

(I spent between forty-five minutes to an hour lifting) and there was no reason to tie up the weight area doing what I could be doing elsewhere.

These four workouts are a bit more intense on each muscle group which encourages muscle growth due to TUT - Time Under Tension.

Again, stay strict. Good form, head into it and lots of air in the lungs.

CYCLE 4

Workout 1

MUSCLE GROUP	EXERCISE	SETS	REPS	REST
CHEST	BENCH PRESS	3	8	2-3 MIN
	DUMBELL FLYE	3	10	1-2 MIN
	INCLINE D/B PRESS	3	10	2-3 MIN
	INCLINE D/B FLYE	3	10	1-2 MIN
TRICEPS	CLOSE GRIP BENCH PRESS	3	10-12	2-3 MIN
	KICKBACKS	3	10	2-3 MIN
	D/B OVERHEAD TRI EXTENSION	3	8-10	2-3 MIN
	SIDE TRICEPS	3	8-10	2-3 MIN

CYCLE 4

Workout 2

MUSCLE GROUP	EXERCISE	SETS	REPS	REST
BACK	BENTOVER B/B ROW	3	8	2-3 MIN
	1-ARM D/B ROW	3	10-12	2-3 MIN
BICEPS	BARBELL/E-Z BAR CURL	3	8-10	2-3 MIN
	INCLINE D/B CURL	3	10	2-3 MIN
	PREACHER CURLS	3	10-12	2-3 MIN
FOREARMS	ZOTTMAN CURLS	3	8-10	2-3 MIN
	WRIST CURL	3	12-15	1-2 MIN
	REVERSE WRIST CURL	3	12-15	1-2 MIN

CYCLE 4

Workout 3

MUSCLE GROUP	EXERCISE	SETS	REPS	REST
LEGS	SQUAT	3	6-8	2-3 MIN
	LEG PRESS	3	10	2-3 MIN
	LEG EXTENSION	3	10-12	1-2 MIN
	LYING LEG CURL	3	10-12	2-3 MIN
CALVES	STANDING CALF RAISE	3	20-25	1-2 MIN
	SEATED CALF RAISE	3	20-25	1-2 MIN

CYCLE 4

Workout 4

MUSCLE GROUP	EXERCISE	SETS	REPS	REST
SHOULDERS	BARBELL SHOULDER PRESS	3	12	2-3 MIN
	D/B LATERAL RAISE	3	12-15	1-2 MIN
	D/B REAR-DELT RAISE	3	12-15	1-2 MIN
TRAPS	BARBELL SHRUG	3	8-10	2-3 MIN
	D/B SHRUG	3	10-12	2-3 MIN

Well, how are you feeling? Great I hope! You have spent the last two months training your body. You've experienced strength and gains in muscle mass. You are now ready to move forward and vary the exercises you do relative to the muscle group you want to work.

Personally, after my first few months of training with the above workouts I was eager to add more exercises, more sets, more reps and less rest time between sets. Growth hormone levels rise when there is less rest between sets which encourages greater muscle growth as well as intensifies fat loss due to accelerated cardio performance.

When you lift, it is never a bad idea to work out with a training partner. They will act as a 'spotter' meaning when they spot that you're in trouble they come to your rescue! At Schuylkill I preferred to work out alone. As I said there were other guys at the weight asylum but in their own "cards" – groups. A card could be up to four guys and having my own card I could bring in a few guys if I wanted. Every now and then I trained guys, as I wrote, but my alone time was precious to me. Knowing there was someone around anyway if I did get into trouble enabled me to train alone.

Use dumbbells and barbells early in the workout because they are more difficult to control and need to be tackled while you're still fresh.

As I mentioned, we didn't have machines at the prison, but as you are training at a gym you most likely do. Use the machines in the middle or end of your workout.

Keeping a journal will help you long term, as now you will see in writing the progress you've made, but it is most useful short-term. You will want to look back to the previous muscle group workout for guidance on your next workout with that group. Write down your diet, a PR- a personal record (which you'll have more and more of) your cardio work, what seemed to work during that workout. Anything you can do to track your progress will help you enormously.

You'll notice that 'down' days – those days you're depressed – will turn around when you work out. Exercise is known to boost your body's endorphins – "ease the pain" proteins generally found in a person's brain – and is also a distraction to a feeling of just feeling bad. The American Journal of Preventive Medicine reviewed thirty different studies and concluded that even low levels of exercise (usually meaning less than 150 minutes per week) may help prevent depression.

Lifting weights can be tough yet very rewarding. Maybe you're familiar with the saying "The best part of working out is when it's over" and while that may hold true every now and then, there is enormous satisfaction performing moves you were not able to do previously with a weight you never thought you'd lift. The most important thing to remember is to maintain good form. If you try to lift too heavy your body lets you know immediately because your form suffers. While you may be able to move the weight somewhat, if you're not going to parallel (on a squat for instance) or starting the next rep of a Military Press below the chin for example you're not really benefiting.

There are specialized training techniques known as Partial Reps, Super Sets, and Drop Sets to name a few, which will help breakthrough sticking points and plateaus and we'll discuss them later.

If you're like most of us the one, single-most one exercise that we'll do most anything to avoid doesn't even involve weights. Or barbells. Or dumbbells. It's abdominal work!

There is no easy way to train the abs. No cute little moves to make the pain go away. However when each and every one of us think of being fit, we think of a flat stomach. There are four main muscles that are found in the abdominals: The Rectus Abdominis, Internal Obliques, External Obliques and The Transverse Abdominis—and to properly train you must hit each one of them.

Known as fundamental exercises, ab work will positively assist you in performing squats, deadlifts and bent over rows. This is due to the ability of the core – which abdominals are a dominant part of – to provide pressure that supports the spine from giving way and falling forward during an exercise.

Ab work can be done along with a regular workout so long as you do them last. Incorporating my ab work during my cardio workout early in the day allowed me five hours of recovery before my weight-lifting routine began. After I returned home, I continued this pattern of performing my abdominal work in the morning. Again, if you decide to work the abs in conjunction with weight training, wait to perform them last.

There are several abdominal exercises that can greatly assist you in building the midsection of your body into a formidable body amour. We will also address them a bit later.

As I continued to train after those first few months, I began to vary the exercises I would use to hit a particular muscle group. I would workout with the same routine for a few months and then use another specific exercise for that body part.

It is highly recommended that you follow a structured training schedule that includes what's known as *Recovery Periods.*

Every six weeks (or when needed) lower the weights you're using by 50 percent. This allows the muscles, tendons and ligaments to somewhat recover. Every twelve weeks take one full week off. However continue to do cardio—biking, rowing, walking, anything that will raise your heartbeat rate for a period of time. Taking a week from lifting will give your body an opportunity to repair itself. Take that time to plan your workouts for the ensuing twelve weeks.

A note of full disclosure: Although I am advising taking a full week off after twelve weeks, that was a recommendation that I – actually most – of us in lock-up, didn't follow. Since the rec yard was always a target of disciplinary action we knew we needed to take advantage of lifting while we were able to. All too often there would be an announcement that made the cardio room and weight pit off limits. We worked hard while we could.

Keep in mind that you don't need to train six days a week. You don't grow in the gym, you grow between workouts. At rest, at home.

Since my workouts changed often it wouldn't be practical to outline each of them here, but I will share a workout schedule that I used many times over those years in the pound.

MONDAY

MUSCLE GROUP	EXERCISE	SETS	REPS	REST
SHOULDERS	SEATED D/B SHOULDER PRESS	4	12	1 MIN
	SEATED LATERAL RAISE	4	12	45 SEC
	SEATED REAR DELTOID RAISE	4	12	45 SEC
	STANDING MILITARY PRESS	4	15-20	1-2 MIN
	LANDMINES	4	12	1 MIN

TUESDAY

MUSCLE GROUP	EXERCISE	SETS	REPS	REST
LEGS	LEG PRESS	4	15	1-2 MIN
	HACK SQUATS	4	12	1-2 MIN
	SQUATS	5	5	1-2 MIN
	STANDING CALF RAISE	3	15-25	1 MIN

WEDNESDAY

MUSCLE GROUP	EXERCISE	SETS	REPS	REST
CHEST	FLAT BENCH D/B PRESS	4	12-15	1 MIN
	FLAT BENCH D/B FLYE	4	12	1 MIN
	INCLINE D/B PRESS	4	12	1-2 MIN
	INCLINE D/B FLYE	4	12	1-2 MIN
	INCLINE OVERHEAD PULLOVER	4	12	1-2 MIN

THURSDAY

MUSCLE GROUP	EXERCISE	SETS	REPS	REST
BICEPS	EZ BAR PREACHER CURLS	4	15-20	1-2 MIN
	ALTERNATING HAMMER CURLS	4	12	1 MIN
TRICEPS	OVERHEAD TRICEPS	4	12	1 MIN
	KICK BACKS	4	15	45 SEC
	SIDE TRICEPS	4	12	1 MIN
FOREARMS	WRIST CURLS	4	20	1 MIN
	REVERSE WRIST CURLS	4	20	1 MIN

FRIDAY

MUSCLE GROUP	EXERCISE	SETS	REPS	REST
BACK	1-ARM D/B ROW	4	12	1 MIN
	UPRIGHT B/B ROW	4	10-12	1 MIN
	BENT OVER B/B ROW	4	12	1 MIN
	DEADLIFTS	3	10,8,6	3 MIN
TRAPS	D/B SHRUG	3	15-25	1 MIN

As you can see, I worked one individual body part per day. Since those of us working out not only needed to stay out of each other's way we had to make adjustments to what muscle groups we combined. For example, Thursdays were arm days – a pull day – for me, yet I had to combine my triceps — a push exercise — with my arm workout. Being

147

respectful to each other's routine was the only way we could get our lifting in.

I used a variety of exercises to work a particular muscle group (which I break down by muscle group in Appendix A) and usually adjusted the workout routine somewhat every three months.

Although I usually performed four sets of a particular exercise there is a strong argument to be made to do as few as three sets. Frankly, four sets worked for me and the general consensus among Fitness Trainers is a scheme of 3-4 sets of an exercise is optimal. The 'sweet spot' as it were, of reps is in the 8-12 rage. This range recruits the fast twitch motor units and elevates both testosterone and growth hormone levels.

Compound movements — also known as multi-joint exercises — engage multiple groups of large muscles. Compound movements are known to release anabolic (growth) hormones as well. [19]

Compound movements include squats, deadlifts, bench presses and T-bar rows, dips, lat pulls, decline bench press, dumbbell dress, pull-ups/chin-ups and any type of row.

Since my cardio workouts were in the early morning, before I ate anything for the day (taking advantage of first burning fat as opposed to carbs) I was recovered sufficiently by mid-afternoon when I lifted.

My ab work included crunches, flutter kicks, reverse crunches, side bends, knee raises and planks (these I incorporated in my yoga movements), which I performed six days per week. Planks were done twice per week.

The abdominal fibers are postural muscles which assists you in maintaining an upright posture throughout the day. Because of this the abs respond well to frequent training.

An expanded list of abdominal exercises can be found in Appendix B. As we did not have machines available as I said, I did not include the exercises that are performed with them however you should incorporate cables, Smith machines, Pec Decks and the like in your training. For instance, cable crunches allow you to add weight to an ab workout in place of body weight only.

You'll also find a variety of exercises, even "novel" ones, in health and fitness websites and magazines, many of which can really help reach those "tuff to train" spots as well as guide you in overcoming plateaus.

A word of caution though – proceed guardedly with unique or unusual exercises. At times you may become aware of a lifting move that you've never been aware of. If your gut feeling urges you not to do it – *Don't!* Some of these moves are proposed to very experienced weight-lifters. Allow me to share a story…

Perhaps you're familiar with a move known as a Hackenschmidt Squat? NO? A Hackenschmidt Squat is basically a deadlift with the barbell placed behind the legs. As in a traditional deadlift (where the bar is in the front of the legs) the back is kept straight and the barbell is lifted using the heels to push through.

One of the gangsters on the compound – 6'4 and 300+ pounds – decided one day that this would be the time to show off his strength in front of his homies. With 315 pounds of pig iron in his grip behind him he slowly lifted the bar from the floor to about mid hamstring at which point he felt something pop in his lower back! The weight fell to the floor at the same moment he did.

Now prison is no place to get sick. The medical staff usually is hard of hearing when it comes to inmate complaints. I personally experienced such when I nearly lost sight in my left eye due to detached retina as you'll recall. When it comes to a sports injury however medical goes deaf. Unless a bone has punctured the skin or an Achilles tendon has rolled up behind the knee, you're on your own. As was our hero. For months (that *is* plural) the only way he could maneuver was by lying prone on a pushcart as he was rolled around the yard by a few of his boys.

There are numerous odd lift exercises – the Steinborn Lift, The Continental clean-and-jerk, and The Arthur to name just a few – that can be dangerous. Perhaps even catastrophic. Be careful and be sensible.

As you advance in training your body – both muscles and your central nervous system – you may find some additional methods known as "Intensity Techniques" helpful with that. These include:

Supersets

These are two distinct and different exercises done with no more than ten seconds rest between. These assist in building up weak areas or resting one body part (if you are exercising two entirely different parts) or exhausting the same muscle group (if working the same part). Supersets are also great cardio work due to the continual movements of your body performing the movement.

Partial Reps

Every exercise you perform (if done correctly) involves what's known as ROM - Range of Motion. Partial reps are just that - short of ROM but allows you to fatigue the fibers of that specific muscle which assists in further growing that muscle. Do not make it a practice to continually perform partial reps however. Always use proper form with ROM, using partial reps occasionally.

Rest-Pause Sets

After reaching failure on your exercise, you rest for ten to fifteen seconds and go again to failure *with the same weight.* Reasonably you will probably not be able to perform the same amount of reps. For instance your first set you performed twelve reps, the second six to eight, the third set four to five. Do no more than three sets of rest-pauses. You'll see results within a few weeks through more endurance and greater musculature on the area worked.

Giant Set

This technique works best with multiple exercises for one body part. Giant sets are performed by completing sets without resting between them. For example, four sets of ten reps in the bench press, then going directly to flat bench dumbbell presses, there to incline dumbbell presses, then four sets of ten reps for an incline dumbbell fly. This is an exhausting workout that will leave nothing on the table.

Dropsets

This technique is very popular with cons for some reason. As I pointed out earlier the weight pile was organized into 'cards'—two to four guys worked out together. Dropsets are performed to failure then the weight is dropped down (by a guy on each side of the lifter) by 20 percent where another set of reps are done. Once again, the weight is dropped another 20 percent or so and another set is performed.

As I worked out alone, I performed drop sets with dumbbells where I could grab them quickly as I progressed downward. I found three sets of ten to twelve reps worked best for me.

Forced Reps

This technique requires a training partner. After reaching failure your partner will help you lift the weight – sometimes with a barbell at other times dumbbells - with your spotter behind you assisting you by placing his hands under your triceps (as in a dumbbell shoulder press for example) and helping you lift the weight. The spotter should not do the work, only slightly assisting the lift for another two or three reps which should be doable. This was another popular technique used behind the razor wire.

Negatives

The general consensus among many is that lifting the weight, known as a concentric move, builds muscle. Actually it's the "eccentric" portion of the repetition that assists in increasing strength and muscle growth as well. Instead of "weightlifting" we would be correct in

152

referring to weight workouts as "weight resisting". Withstanding the effect of gravity on the weight is the primary cause of muscle soreness over a period of days following a workout.

This is another technique that will require a training partner as they will assist you in lifting the weight (known as the positive portion of the move) while you slowly lower the weight counting to three as you do. Your partner will continue to assist you during your set in the same manner. They will also 'spot' you in case your muscles give out to prevent an injury.

Negatives will significantly add to muscle mass as well as great confidence when you lift on your own.

These methods are what someone serious about packing on muscle will perform. These techniques are great for overcoming sticking points and plateaus but doing more than a few of them in a single workout is not recommended as they are extremely demanding on the muscles as well as your nervous system. Personally, I devoted a specific workout periodically to perform these methods on a particular muscle group but, again, only a couple of them at any one workout.

Before we leave the topic of techniques to help you gain strength and size, one method that I used consistently on Push and Pull exercises were wrist wraps. Wrist wraps will give your wrists extra support during heavy weightlifting sessions. They will steady the wrists and also relieves pressure on them as well as absorbing the load instead of the elbows during overhead presses.

If you decide to use upper-arm wraps they will help to reduce the flow of blood to the muscles in the upper arms. This constriction, research has found, can increase the stores of growth hormone by 290%!

As I was mentally preparing to report to prison, I had the opportunity to speak to a business acquaintance, Larry, who years earlier had done time for a tax case. Desperate to learn anything I could about prison I asked Larry what I should expect. Afterwards he wrapped up our conversation with this advice: "You do the time, don't let the time do you."

I recall thinking "That's a weird statement. What does that even mean?" After being locked up for a few months I understood what he meant.

Prison is slow time. It is a thief that steals hopes, dreams, and years. It eats away at a man's soul and invites a loathing, a sense of worthlessness that can become a part of you for the rest of your life.

If you allow it.

A lot of cons do their time hustling, contradicting authority, and irritating others. Some do nothing, lying around without ambition. A few take the time to improve themselves through classes— GED, HVAC, Solar and Culinary Arts to name a few.

I took whatever classes were offered and I taught classes as well. In addition, I mentored the new guys, gave piano lessons, tutored, organized summer and Christmas music programs and was very involved in our Christian ministry. I was the proverbial rolling stone in lock-up, that gathered no moss. I made sure I managed my time.

I did not have the luxury if that's the word, of feeling sorry for myself. I never lost consciousness of the fact that I was responsible to dozens of investors in my company that needed to be repaid after my time with the BOP was over. It would be on me, on my shoulders alone to do so. In order to accomplish that I had to make a commitment to excellence. To be the best I could be in every area of my life.

I knew my health, my stamina, and my strength needed to transcend anything I once knew. I needed to not only improve, but surpass, to somehow turn back the hands of time and commandeer the energy, vitality, and sturdiness of a twenty-one-year-old man.

It was in my private time, after my work in the chapel was complete, and between studying and writing that I focused on building my personal physical armor.

The following is the cardio, the core work and the body weight training that - and I say this humbly - brought me there.

Use common sense, keep in mind that it took me nearly nine years to reach the ensuing workouts. Although I experimented with a number of specific cardio, core, body weight and yogic exercises moves, I found these to be the most effective - for me. I encourage you to consider these disciplines as a source from which you'll discover through experimentation, dedication and determination, what will work the most effectively for you.

CARDIO

CARDIO IS THE DEVIL

-Unknown

METHOD   **DURATION**

ROWING MACHINE   15 MINUTES

NOTES:

HIIT – 45 seconds of steady rowing (qualifying as 'rest'),   15 seconds of intense rowing

ELLIPTICAL   15 MINUTES

NOTES:

HIIT – 45 seconds of steady walking, 15 seconds of intense running

STATIONARY BIKE   15 MINUTES

NOTES:

HIIT – 45 seconds of steady pedaling, 15 seconds of intense
pedaling. Final 4 minutes switch to TABATA PROTOCOL: 20 seconds
intense pedaling, 10 seconds of steady pedaling.

I began my morning workout performing cardio training first. I
found the rowing machine an effective all-inclusive exercise to start
with. The rowing machine is not only an outstanding cardio trainer but is
an exceptional exercise that also targets the chest, shoulders, biceps, back
and legs.

Most rowing machines are equipped with various levels of
tension, usually from 1 to 10. Personally, I remained at level 10 to
complete the 15-minute cycle of HIIT. After 15 minutes I found an
increase in my heartbeat per minute (BPM) of 40% to 98 BPM (My
personal resting heartbeat being approximately 58).

I then moved to the Elliptical machine performing another 15
minutes of HIIT. This workout increased my BPM another 20% to 124+
within 8-10 minutes and remaining there for the duration of the Elliptical
work.

To complete the cardio circuit, I moved to the stationary bike
again performing HIIT but concluding the stationary bike workout with 4
minutes of the TABATA Protocol. My BPM varied between 124 and 130
at this point.

I was very aware of the importance of maintaining an effective
cardio workout. In order to arrest the heart attack, I experienced in 2008

(when I was 54 years old) the Cardiologist inserted stents into three of my arteries including one in my Aorta which had a 90% blockage! Consequently, I spent a considerable amount of time on Cardio work as you can see.

Although you're likely thinking "he had the time" - and certainly I had "a lot of time" - please keep in mind that recalls, counts, shakedowns and lockdowns we're so frequent that I worked like an animal when I had the opportunity. Unfortunately, as I mentioned earlier, our machines were prone to breakdowns due to their age and excessive use. In the slammer you get the work in when you can - a concept I carry with me even now.

If you have been working out but noticing fewer positive results you may be overtraining. Generally cardio overtraining is caused by long, continuous workouts. Feeling fatigue can be a sign of cellular exhaustion if indeed you are training like this. An effective remedy is performing short bursts of intense exercise - HIIT. Performing intense interval training has the ability to not only strengthen the heart muscle but to fight conditions like Osteoporosis (thinning of the bones) and Sarcopenia (muscle wasting) as well.

In the free world it's easy to blow off exercising. I know - I did it for years. Work, kid's baseball and football games. Work. Family commitments. Work. Keeping up a home. And more work.

The University of Cambridge conducted research some years back comparing BMI (body mass index), waist size and the physical activity levels of over 330,000 people over a 12-year span. *What they found is that the lack of physical activity was responsible for twice as many deaths as obesity!*

Ulf Ekelund, the study's author observed that "Physical activity has positive effects on blood pressure, glucose metabolism, and insulin sensitivity, regardless of being overweight." He went on to say "Exercise – and the more the better, is one of the best medical treatments you can get."

If you find yourself short on time and can't get a good workout in *FOR A VALID REASON,* consider the 5-minute workout for one of the following:

EXERCISE	CALORIES BURNED
PUSH-UPS OR PULL-UPS	51
JOGGING	53
SWINGING A KETTLEBELL	63
JUMPING ROPE	79

Let's be honest - life has a habit of getting in the way of best intentions, but *exercising is for you*! One of the most effective remedies for depression (and I know this to be true through years in prison) is intense HIIT. 'Preventive Medicine' found in research they did, a connection between increased serotonin (a neurotransmitter which causes a narrowing of the interior diameter of the blood vessels) levels and aerobic and muscle-strengthening exercise.

High Intensity Interval Training is, if nothing else, an explosive, endurance-building program of exercise. You'll recall when I mentioned how some of the strongest guys on the block were cardio weak and stamina hindered? These types of workouts are meant to prevent you from running out of gas - whether at the company softball game or an attempted take-down in the yard.

Cardio work will get you shredded and fit. Cardio work - real, dedicated and resolute cardio work - has the ability to not only add years to your life but ensure that those years are of the highest quality.

BODY WEIGHT

EXERCISE	SETS	REPS	REST
PUSHUPS	6	F	1 MIN

NOTES:

> Keeping your torso in a straight line, feet together, hands shoulder-width (or wider if you prefer) apart and head slightly looking forward, perform as many reps as possible in each of 6 sets, resting for 1 minute between sets.

EXERCISE	SETS	REPS	REST
CRUNCHES	10	F	1 MIN

NOTES:

> Crunches can be performed with feet flat on the floor or raised with knees slightly bent. Cradle your head (as opposed to 'pulling' your head and neck) while raising your upper torso. Hold the top position for a moment and, if possible, a bit longer.

EXERCISE	SETS	REPS	REST
FLUTTER KICK	3	<15	1 MIN

NOTES:

Lie flat on your back, hands behind your head. With legs extended straight (no bend in the knees) raise them 6-10 inches of the floor. Use a 10-count, kicking the feet up and down with a controlled movement. Lower and repeat. Work up to 15 reps.

EXERCISE	SETS	REPS	REST
KNEE RAISE	4	<25	1 MIN

NOTES:

KNEE RAISES are easily performed on a workout bench or any flat surface. Using your hands as support on either side of your sitting position, raise the knees high, parallel or a bit higher, to the floor. Perform 4 sets working up to 25 reps.

EXERCISE	SETS	REPS	REST
DIPS	5	<20	1 MIN

NOTES:

Using a Dip Bar, lower yourself to a ninety-degree angle at your elbows. Return to the full extension. Your feet should be extended in the air, usually knees slightly bent. If a Dip Bar is not available any flat and stable surface can suffice, in which case your legs are extended straight, heels on the floor, hands on either side, palms flat, hands facing away from you. Perform 5 sets working up to 20 reps. To prevent possible shoulder issues, do not place your hands behind your back.

EXERCISE	SETS	REPS	REST
NECK RAISES	3	> 40	1 MIN

NOTES

Every guy who has been in the system for a while and who is into muscle training can spot someone who is the real deal or a wannabe. The wannabe is the one who trains the showy stuff – biceps and maybe chest. Throw a pair of shorts on them and you can tell they are allergic to the squat rack as well. The dead give-away though is a guy's neck. Most never even think about working the neck but that is where the bad boys differ. They train where others don't, so they are always combat ready.

There are three basic moves for a strong neck, but you must *use common sense* doing them. Especially starting out. This is a long-game exercise. Give it 12 months though and you will continue to get fitted with ever larger collars.

Lying on your back, begin with one to five reps each: 1) lift the head to the chest. 2) Raise the head again and look to the right. Repeat on the left. 3) Raise the head, touch the right ear to the right shoulder. Repeat on the left. This is one set. You want to aim for three sets. Continue to increase the reps until you reach 40 on each move. Do this progressively. Add a few more every few weeks. It will likely take 12 months or more to reach 40 but hang in there. I incorporate these into my work out twice a week. Doing deadlifts, shrugs, upright rows and power cleans are a great way to add bulk to the neck and the traps as well.

POSTURE

Before the judge threw away the key on me, my posture was pretty poor. Maybe my increasing weight had something to do with it, (to say nothing of feeling beat down after I caught my case) but this was an adjustment that I consciously worked on. Although there is not a particular "exercise" for posture, there is a stance that will enormously help improve someone's posture. Stand against a wall – heels, glutes, elbows, shoulders and head touching the wall. This needs to be a wall without base molding so as to allow everything in strict alignment. Stand straight for sixty seconds. Close your eyes for a portion of that time and really "feel" the state of your frame. Become part of it. Do this at least once a day. I promise you will see an improvement in a short amount of time in not only your stance but your walk as well. Don't bother saying *"I'm too old!"* I'm probably older than you!! This works.

163

Behind the fence every item has a use. A Q-tip bag becomes a zip lock bag to hold tweezers, nail clippers and scissors. A cracker box becomes a shelf in a locker. A garbage bag becomes a cooking container and your body becomes workout equipment.

As a stand-alone workout program or in combination with weight training, using the heft of your body will greatly assist in not only gaining strength and endurance but will help you acquire a firm, lean and chiseled appearance. Body weight moves can be done most anywhere which makes them a convenient alternative if you can't get to the gym.

As I looked back in my journal, I was reminded again how pathetically out of shape I entered prison. I began to do (*attempt* would be a more accurate word) body weight moves after a few months of focusing on weight loss through Cardio work. "6/20/12 - 3 sets of push-ups, 3 reps per set" My notes were as follows *"Hard, and Form Bad"* My notes on my first attempt at crunches in years, which took place a few days later on June 29th, reads "2 sets - 3 reps on Set 1, 5 reps on set 2" As you can see, I had my work cut out for me!

As the years passed, along with my cardio workout I incorporated the body weight exercises above 6 days a week - 10 sets of 50 crunches per workout, 3 sets of Flutter kicks for 15 reps, reverse crunches – 3 sets of 20 reps as well as push-ups.

I performed push-ups daily - 6 sets of 50 except on Friday when I did 40 sets of 25. I used the first Friday of every month to complete 60 sets of 25 reps. After I performed these multiple sets the first time I attempted them, I could not get my head around to not continue to do them. It would feel like I was allowing myself to go backwards. I was not – *and will never* – allow that to ever happen!

On the days I performed multiple sets of 25 push-ups I rested 30 seconds between sets otherwise I paused a full minute.

As you can see, I did not include pull-ups or chin-ups in my workouts. Despite several enthusiastic attempts over the years, I was unable to pull my body up due to the searing pain in my left shoulder. Years ago when I was lifting, I incorporated Behind-the-Neck shoulder presses - a move I have since learned can cause real damage to the shoulders. Knowing what I know now I strongly suggest *not* doing them. During my time inside I attributed the pain I was experiencing in my shoulder to perhaps a torn Rotator cuff. It made sense since the pain was localized. When I finally came home, I was examined by an Orthopedist. What he found was not a torn R. C. but arthritis! He confirmed that doing Behind-the-Neck presses directly contributed to my shoulder dilemma. No problem, I just take it into consideration and work around it!

That said I encourage you to include pull-ups and chin-ups in your workout routine. No exercise can build a tapered V-shaped back like these movements. Lat pulldowns do come in a *very* close second. Begin with three sets, one or two reps. You will know when to increase the reps. Make sure to constantly challenge yourself.

After I completed my Cardio and body weight exercises, I finished my workout performing Yoga.

Yoga is a system of mental and physical exercise that has been practiced for thousands of years. The word Yoga comes to us from the Sanskrit (the classical language of India) and means "Union".

Incorporating Yoga into your workouts will indeed take the union of body, mind and spirit, but the benefits of integrating the strength and flexibility found from the postures – known as "Asana's" – will build a formidable and sturdy core.

The practice sequence I used allowed me to develop a solid foundation that assisted me in my other workouts.

If it was possible to find inner solitude inside the nuthouse otherwise known as Federal Prison, I was able to do so through not only meditation but my cardio, weight training and yoga practice as well.

If you are new to the journey of yoga the following sequence will allow you to gently step into the graceful world of this ancient practice. Although, as in so much of life, it will take time and patience before you'll feel confident, the practice of yoga will become a source, a well really, of not only strength and flexibility but of peace and internal serenity. You will find yoga another source of meditation as well.

YOGA

Although here in the West, Yoga poses are rarely referred to by their Sanskrit names, I thought it helpful to include them for clarity.

Since these poses should be viewed instead of read, I am listing only the benefits associated with each of them. I encourage you to view these Asana's online for the correct posture, stance and movement of them. Better by far would be to study with a Certified Yoga Instructor.

Including Yoga in your schedule will significantly strengthen your core muscles as well as provide you with a serene mindfulness while you are doing so as I pointed out

PLANKS

CHATARANGA DANDASANA

This pose strengthens the abdominals especially, also the shoulder, spine, quads and chest.

This is a form that produces force throughout the body, establishing stabilization of the core. Work up to holding this position for one minute with a sixty-second pause between poses. Set a longer-range goal of three minutes.

If there is only one asana you should perform, this is the one.

SIDE PLANKS

VASISTHASANA

This pose strengthens the oblique muscles directly but also targets the shoulders, hips and legs. The spine is directly affected, and this asana is a bit more challenging than the plank as you will be balancing first on one side then the other. Work up to holding this pose for 30 seconds per side.

KNEE TO CHEST POSE

APANASANA

Affects the lower back by stretching the spine. Also stretches the glutes and quads. Hold for one minute (8 to 10 breaths)

SPINE TWIST

SUPTA MATSYENDRAIANA

The spine twist allows for a release in the hips as well as opens the shoulders. The glutes are stretched as is the entire spine. This pose also creates space between the vertebrates as you may feel - and possibly hear. Hold for one minute (8 to 10 breaths)

CAT COW (VARIATION)

UPAVISTHA BITILASANA MARJARYASANA

Strengthens the spine and neck as well as stretching them. The CAT COW asana also stretches the hips, abdomen and back muscles. This pose is also referred to as the "Bird Dog", due to the arm and leg movements and extensions of both. Work up to ten sets of five seconds each side.

LOCUST POSE

SALABHASANA

This asana *greatly* strengthens the muscles of the spine, glutes and the backs of the arms and legs. It also stretches the shoulders, chest, abdomen and thighs. This posture can help improve your posture as well. Also known as the "Superman" pose. Work up to ten sets holding from three to five seconds.

UPWARD DOG

URDHVA MUKHA SVANASANA

This pose stretches the abdominal muscles as well as the chest and spine. It assists in strengthening the arms and shoulders. Also work up to ten sets holding the position from three to five seconds. Similar to a push-up, the difference is that your entire lower torso remains on the ground.

CHILD'S POSE

BALASANA

This is a gentle resting pose that stretches the lower back, hips, thighs, knees and ankles. It relaxes the spine, shoulder and neck as well increasing the blood circulation to the head which has been known to relieve headaches. This is a great stand-alone pose as it alleviates stress, fatigue and tension. Hold the Child's pose for one minute although you may find yourself holding it longer due its relaxing effect on your entire body. Here you are on your knees, face down, arms outstretched.

DOWNWARD DOG

ADHO MUKHA SVANASANA

This asana strengthens the arms and legs while stretching the shoulders, hamstrings, calves, arches and hands. This very familiar pose can also prevent osteoporosis. Hold for one minute (8 to 10 breaths).

STANDING FORWARD BEND

UTTANASANA

The hips, hamstrings and calves are stretched in this pose while strengthening the thighs and knees. Hold for one minute (8 to 10 breaths).

WIDE LEG STANDING FORWARD BEND

PRASARITA PADOTTANASANA

This asana stretches as well as strengthens the hamstrings, calves, hips, lower back, and spine. Due to the position of the arms the shoulders, wrists, forearms and upper back will feel stretched. Hold for one minute (8 to 10 breath).

BRIDGE POSE

SETU BANDMM SARVANGASANA

This pose opens the chest, heart and hip flexor. It stretches the chest, neck, shoulders and spine while simultaneously strengthening the back, glutes, legs and ankles. This is another great core exercise. Hold this asana up to a minute and a half (10 to 12 breaths). While on your back, arms to the side. raise the hips with the feet anchoring your stance.

TREE POSE

VRKASANA

The Tree Pose strengthens the thigh, calves, core and foot muscles. In addition to improving the posture. This asana stretches the inner thighs, groin and shoulders. This is a balance exercise that would be best worked up to a one-minute pose on each side (8 to 10 breaths on each side). Have a sturdy object nearby to touch if needed. This will also assist you if this pose is new to you as it will help to develop the leg muscles. The body constantly makes slight correctional movements so you will likely not be able to stand perfectly still. This is called Dynamic

Balance Movement and results from constant agonist – antagonist muscle contractions. Those muscles – like all exercise - will strengthen over time if you are persistent. This pose will really help with your balance going forward.

EYE OF THE NEEDLE

SUCIRANDHRASANA

This is a movement that stretches the muscles around the hips, lower back and hamstrings. The Eye of the Needle pose also stretches the glutes and quads. This pose is performed by lying on the back ankle over the top of the opposite knee. Work each side. Hold for thirty to sixty seconds (3-10 breaths). *Do not force the stretch, go only as deep as comfortable.*

RECLINING EAGLE POSE

SUPTA GARUDASANA

This asana stretches the arms and shoulders as well as the upper back however this movement is especially beneficial in stretching the hips and pelvis. Hold for one minute (8 to 10 breaths). Lying on the back, cross the leg to the other side.

REVOLVED ABDOMEN POSE

JATHARA PARIVARTANASANA

Another asana that will stretch the arms and shoulders, hips and pelvis but now hitting the abdomen as well. Lift the bended knees to your chest, keeping the shoulder blades on the floor. Tilt the knees to the right holding for one minute and then repeat on the left.

CLEANSING BY FIRE (ALSO KNOWN AS CHURNING)

AGNI SARA DHAUTI

Strengthens the abdominal muscles while toning the pelvis and abdominal regions of the body. Bend over slightly, hands on hips and completely exhale letting all the air out of your lungs. Hold for ten seconds or more if possible. This asana takes getting used to as the breath needs to be controlled. It can also be performed standing up straight. Perform this asana on a *completely empty* stomach.

FISH POSE

MATSYASANA

I personally ended my Yogic asanas with the Fish Pose. This posture opens the neck, chest and the entire Thorax. Allow yourself two to five undisturbed minutes for this pose. On the back you are placing a rolled towel or thin yoga mat directly underneath the spine, arms to the side. Very relaxing as you will feel the release across the chest.

Each of these poses promotes balance, strength and flexibility. Be patient and if you are not able to hold the pose for the suggested amount of time that's fine. Once you've become accustomed to the asana itself you will find yourself holding the pose with proficiency. Possibly even longer if you wish. These poses are suitable for beginners as well as valuable for advanced students.

I found that stretching after my Cardio and bodyweight training greatly benefited my weightlifting a few hours later. Although I carried out my asana practice six days a week, I performed planks and side planks no more than two times per week.

There is an abundance of Yogic poses that are increasingly complicated and advanced – but doable for someone dedicated to the practice. What I've listed here benefited me immensely as I think they will you also.

THROUGH A GLASS DARKLY

As a kid growing up in Western New York, it was not unusual to climb into the car, drive across the Rainbow Bridge and spend the day in Canada.

Living just across the river - the Niagara River separates the two countries - made for a quick and easy ride back then, "Where were you born? How long will you be in Canada? Anything to declare? Have a nice day!" That was it! There was a reason the US/ Canadian crossings were considered the world's friendliest border, and this was but one example. Of course, this was before 9/11 and now in place of a 2-minute delay *a 2-hour wait* is common.

Although a US citizen, my mother had been born in Italy, but I remember my father's answer when asked his birthplace.

The first of three boys, my father was born in Pennsylvania shortly after my grandfather Antonio Iovannisci and my grandmother Anna arrived in the US from the region of Abruzzo, that part of Italy that would remind you of the calf on the Italian boot. When my grandparents were processed on Ellis Island, they were given a new name – Gane.

"Why don't you just tell them you were born in Buffalo?" I asked my father "nobody ever heard of that stupid place you were born!" Despite being one of the kindest and sweetest men I ever knew, I'm shocked, as I look back, that he didn't turn around and swat me!

As the years passed, my mother and father both gone now, I had begun my career in finances and was blessed with a family of my own, and then in turn, we also made those trips to Canada.

After becoming the target of the government someone asked me "Do you want to take off to Italy?" Knowing I had family there. "No!" I said, "When the Feds learn the truth, I'll be fine!"

As time continued to march forward and the investigation continued for years, I began to worry *"My God, what would I do if I really did go to prison?"* As preposterous (at the time anyway) as the thought was, it was too scary to think about (remember what I wrote about visualization!). "The truth will set me free" was the mantra that I clung to back then.

But one day curiosity finally got the better of me *"Where would I go?"* I wondered. I browsed the Justice Department's Website which identified the various facilities in its Bureau of Prison's locations throughout the country. There's a ton!

The closest facilities to Buffalo were in Pennsylvania – McKean, outside of Erie the closest to home, Lewisburg, Allenwood. There were a lot of them. I noticed one more but couldn't pronounce the name - Shukill, Schykill. "I wonder where that one is?" as I hit the icon. I stared at the screen in disbelief, the hair on my arms on end. It was then, at that moment, I knew I was going to prison.

Although charges were yet to be filed against me – indeed it would still be over a year before they were – not only did I know I was going to prison but that I would be incarcerated at Schuylkill. You see, that "stupid place no one ever heard of" where my father was born was Minersville, Pennsylvania – where Federal Correctional Institution Schuylkill (pronounced Skoo-kul by the locals) is located!

It's easy to pass off signs, premonitions, omens and of course "feelings", assuming they're nothing more than coincidences. As humans we are bombarded with so much sensory information that an overload of those 'data-bytes' takes place which routinely fall on deaf ears, or simply ignored. In a busy life how much time does a person really have to analyze – either logically or emotionally – the significance of the message? Unless you have a high sense of discernment (which habitually occurs by maintaining a deeply sincere prayer life) as well as a high degree of patience, you may miss those clues. This "higher sense" must be developed – then relied upon - if you hope to stay unmolested when you're surrounded by random psychopaths – many with body counts.

When I read "Minersville, Pennsylvania" that day, I absorbed the sign – regardless of not wanting it so – of what my future held in store, whether those sensations deliver you from evil intensions behind the fence or walking through a parking ramp, it is in each of our best interests to pay attention to them.

Becoming prison-strong, prison-tough, prison-cut takes focus, commitment and consistency. Mostly however, it takes a strong desire to be in the best shape of your life.

Of course, when your safety is dependent on getting jacked it's an easy call but in the land of the free you have to really want it. But know this – it is in your power to achieve it!

A few final thoughts to keep in mind as you are getting bigger, stronger and more self-assured:

Don't be afraid to mix things up. What I'm saying is – Don't continue to do the same workouts, the same exercises constantly. If you do you will simply stop growing. There are any number of different exercises that can, and do, hit most every muscle group.

Educate yourself with the workout information found online, through lifting magazines or optimally with a Certified Fitness Trainer. The weight training workout that I illustrated previously is but one of a half-dozen I used.

Another thing – Get Mad at the Bar! This means - *Be aggressive when you approach the rack!* Grasp the bar with authority. Know you're going to move the weight. Feel the move in your body before the lift. Visualize clearly you're accomplishing the set!

Although I advise resting one to three minutes between workouts, especially in the beginning phase, more accomplished lifters may want to consider using shorter rests. Personally, I may rest for thirty to sixty seconds – depending on my goal it may be as short as 15 seconds - between sets depending on the muscle group I'm working.

Short pauses between work sets accelerates heart rhythm effecting an efficient cardio workout and will burn additional calories in turn as I've written.

Consider using a weight belt (also known as a lifting belt). Usually made of leather, weight belts assist in stabilizing your torso on heavy lifts. Military presses, squats and deadlifts come to mind here. Contrary to popular belief, weight belts primarily secure the abs rather than the back. If used properly weight belts help grind out great work sets.

Use incentives to blast through a sticking point. My secret, personal incentives, ones that I used for years in lockup were compliments of some former family members.

One liquored-up brother-in-law said to me in front of the family shortly before my sentence "Well Guy, we're sure gonna miss ya!" Nice.

After my sentence was handed down, another one said "Whad'ya gonna do about my sister?" Waiting for him to continue, he said "Your gonna have to divorce her. You're gonna be gone for years!" I was cut to the bone when he said that but man, those two comments were *always* good for another rep or two! Actually, still are!

By the late winter of 2019-2020 as my time was finally winding down, I had been in the Cardio room and weight pile steadily for nearly 7 years plus 2 more when I just had Cardio available. Physically (if not completely emotionally) I was in the best condition of my life. I had constantly reminded myself that my time in lock up needed to be put to the best use possible. I continued my cardio work in the morning, which lasted anywhere from 1 1/2 half to 2 hours per, and weight training for at least one hour every afternoon as I related earlier. Not only did I want to do this, I *NEEDED* to. For me, it kept me focused on something other than being locked up. I saw the results but so did the compound. In the joint you never let your guard down and you never take anything for granted. One unintended consequence of my training was that I wasn't looked on as an 'older guy." What I mean is this – generally – but not always, the older guys, over 50, 55, were considered an easy mark. Feeling they could get away with hassling an older guy, some of the street guys might single out someone to harass or bother. Maybe run their mouth to intimidate them. It usually worked. Although I never looked for problems and I showed respect (a *really big deal* in lockup as I wrote earlier) by my actions, I was not going to be a victim either.

For years it was known that my work ethic was pretty intense so consequently I didn't get a pass for being older. Not that I was in any way interested in anyone on the block assuming that anyway! Although I was not looked on as an easy mark, that didn't mean that once in a while some clown didn't decide to test me. I had more than my share of nose-to-nose confrontations over the years and, truth be told, a bit more intense than that on occasion.

Though my Christian Faith was and is oak strong, I was not *ever* going to allow anyone to take advantage of me or my nature as I once did when I craved the approval of others. I once heard the Evangelist Joyce Meyers say, "Just because you're a Christian, doesn't mean you should be a doormat". Truthfully, I wish I could have heard that much earlier in my life instead of a few months before I went to prison, but her words have made an impact on me then - and now. You see, that soft guy who allowed people to talk down to him, who allowed someone to push their finger into his chest in front of a store full of people, who allowed himself to be barked at in front of a room full of strangers is long gone.

I recalled in the Bible that David, when totally disrespected by Nabal, "girded on his sword" for battle. And although certainly not a

King, I would never again allow myself to ever be disrespected by anyone as well. 1 Samuel 25:13

UNTETHERD

Let the words of my mouth and the meditation of my heart Be acceptable in Your sight O Lord.......

-Psalm 19:14

It was at that point - March of 2020 – when my, and the world's, lives were turned upside down. The COVID-19 pandemic, which had begun in China at the close of 2019 was now ravaging Europe and by early March landed on the shores of America. The powers that be within the Bureau of Prisons decided that the best course of action to prevent the spread of the virus to their 180,000 plus guests would be to cancel all visits which they did in early March of that year. Although each of us inside were disappointed we all agreed that it was for the best. With chronic overcrowding in the nation's prisons, they are, in reality a veritable petri dish of disease and with that concern in mind the BOP put all of its institutions on quarantine on March 31. No movement of any kind on the compound was allowed and each inmate was confined to their block.

Meals were structured to allow small groups to go to the Chow Hall by themselves. This went on for nearly three months until by early June we were finally allowed 2 hours per day, 5 days a week to walk or run the track. Everyone had cabin fever by that point and considering the temperature inside the building hovered in the 80s-90s along with high humidity there was a mass exodus that ran out the doors once we could. The buildings were segregated by different time schedules so not everyone was out at the same time. Church services, Library, Education as well as the cardio room, and weight pile were off limits. The very next day, April 1st, I began my body weight training in my cube. Push-ups, crunches, flutter kicks, reverse crunches, dips and yoga. Cardio consisted of fast paced stair climbing up and down three levels in the housing unit for 15 minutes. All for 6 days a week. Although I saw a decrease in muscle size - nothing can adequately replace hard core lifting - I did what was available to me. Having qualified for the provision in the First Step Act, I was schedule to leave at the end of July so wanting to at least maintain whatever I could, I really stepped it up during these workouts. As I counted the days down to my release, now just a few weeks away, I got hit by another unexpected roadblock and this one right in the solar plexus.

By the summer 2020, the second wave of the virus was overtaking the country so the deep thinkers at the BOP decided that anyone being released after July 15th needed an additional dose of quarantine. On the 14th I was informed that the following day - July 15th - I would be brought to the Medium Security Prison facility across the road and serve my remaining time locked in a cell 24/7. During my previous transfers I was also thrown in a cell, but in these instances, I could come and go during the day, locked in only at night. Now I was to be locked in around the clock. For 16 days! Although over the years inside I learned to expect the unexpected (while doing my best not to become institutionalized) you're never quite prepared to be cast into a tiny 11x7 cloister with someone else.

Fortunately, I knew Mark from the camp, a Chinese guy from NYC, but I can tell you - nothing is more degrading, in addition to losing your dignity and your privacy as well, then to be forced to live in conditions like that. And this after already being "quarantined" for nearly 4 months! Thankfully - for both of us, Mark left to go home after 8 days, and I was alone for another 8. Mark was great though and he gave me my space to work out in the cell.

Not even sometimes, but usually, we get so caught up with our own thinking of the way things should be, how they should go, that we neglect to let go and let God. To just totally surrender to His will. Once I was alone in that hot and humid cell for a few days I realized - once again - that He had my back.

Now everything was quiet. Other than having my temperature taken twice a day by the prison medical staff and being fed three times a day (all of this done through the small aperture in the otherwise locked three-inch steel door) there was no more noise. No screaming, no arguments, no swearing, no talking in the middle of the night without regard for anyone. Nothing. Just silence. The author Father Thomas Keating once wrote "Silence is God's first language. Everything else is a poor translation." And it was there, finally alone, that I felt His complete presence.

Answers to questions I had long forgotten began to be given. Wisdom on subjects I hadn't thought of for many years - and on ones I never considered - began to appear. Hurts, betrayals, the lies told about me by others to exonerate themselves, and the bitterness I felt over a dozen years all disappeared. Being locked up, quarantined was nothing I wanted nor ever wished for but, I am so thankful for it. Now, I knew I could go home with a clean heart, with malice toward none, and begin the process of repaying WaterMark's investors.

There is an old adage I recall: "When you're going through hell - keep going." That's the time you must dig down deep, to crawl deeply into your very soul and face your fears head-on.

Never lose sight of the truth that you are a treasure of our Creator, a child of the living God and if God is for you, who can possibly be against you?

Nothing 'just' happens in our lives regardless of the challenges, the heartbreaks or the losses. And if you find that those who you trusted and those who you loved gave up on you - never, ever give up on yourself. Never! Keep fighting the good fight, keep running the race, keep believing in yourself and make your darkest hour your defining moment.

APPENDIX A

I routinely varied my workouts to include exercises that would tax a specific muscle group.

If you continue to do the same moves during every workout you will plateau. Introducing new challenges to a muscle will assist you in muscle growth as well as avoiding boredom. Below are the power moves that will enhance your lifting routine as well as suggestions for sets, reps and rest periods.

These are NOT to be done at the same time! These are the specific exercises that focus on *that particular muscle group* named.

MUSCLE GROUP	EXERCISE	SETS	REPS	REST
LEGS	SQUATS	3-4	5	1-2 MIN
	LEG PRESS	3-4	15	1-2 MIN
	LYING LEG CURLS	4	10	1-2 MIN
	HACK SQUATS	4	10-12	1-2 MIN
	ROMANIAN DEAD LIFTS	4	10-8-6	1-2 MIN
	WALKING LUNGES	3	6-8	1-2 MIN
	REVERSE HAMSTRING			
	EXTENSION	4	F	3 MIN
CALVES	STANDING CALF RAISE	3	15-25	1 MIN
	SEATED CALF RAISE			

MUSCLE GROUP	EXERCISE	SETS	REPS	REST
BICEPS	BARBELL CURLS	3	8-10	1-2 MIN
	PREACHER CURLS	3-4	15-20	1-2 MIN
	INCLINE D/B CURLS	3	8-10	1-2 MIN
	ALTERNATING HAMMER CURLS	3-4	10-12	1-2 MIN
	CONCENTRATION CURLS	3	8-10	1-2 MIN
	SEATED D/B CURLS	3	8-10	1-2 MIN
	STANDING ALTERNATING			
	D/B CURLS	3	10-12	1-2 MIN
FOREARMS	WRIST CURL	4	20	1 MIN
	REVERSE WRIST CURL	4	20	1 MIN

MUSCLE GROUP	EXERCISE	SETS	REPS	REST
CHEST	BENCH PRESS	4	6-8	1-2 MIN
	FLAT BENCH D/B PRESS	4	10-12	1 MIN
	FLAT BENCH D/B FLYE	3-4	10-12	1 MIN
	INCLINE BARBEL PRESS	4	8-12	1-2 MIN
	D/B INCLINE PRESS	3-4	10-12	1-2 MIN
	D/B INCLINE FLYE	3-4	10	1-2 MIN
	D/B INCLINE HAMMER CURL	3	10	1-2 MIN
TRICEPS	CLOSE GRIP BENCH PRESS	3	6-8	1-2 MIN
	D/B OVERHEAD TRICEP	3	8-10	1-2 MIN
	D/B OVERHEAD TRICEP PULLOVER	3-4	10-12	1-2 MIN
	D/B SIDE TRICEP HAMMER	3-4	8-10	1-2 MIN

MUSCLE GROUP	EXERCISE	SETS	REPS	REST
SHOULDERS	SEATED B/B SHOULDER PRESS	3-4	10-12	1-2 MIN
	SEATED D/B LATERAL RAISE	4	10-12	1-2 MIN
	SEATED D/B REAR DELT RAISE	4	10-12	1-2 MIN
	SEATED D/B FRONT RAISE	4	10-12	1-2 MIN
	STANDING D/B OVERHEAD PRESS	4	6-8	1 MIN
	STANDING D/B LATERAL RAISE	4	8-10	1-2 MIN
	STANDING D/B REAR DELT RAISE	4	8-10	1-2 MIN
	STANDING D/B FRONT RAISE	4	8-10	1-2 MIN
	BARBELL UPRIGHT ROW	3	8-10	1-2 MIN
	BARBELL INCLINE FRONT RAISE	3	10	1-2 MIN
	ARNOLD PRESS	4	8-10	1-2 MIN
	MILITARY PRESS	4	10-12	1-2 MIN
	LEANING D/B LATERAL RAISE	4	8	1-2 MIN
TRAPS	BARBELL SHRUG	4	6-8	1 MIN
	DUMBBELL SHRUG	4	8-10	1 MIN

I have addressed HIIT throughout these pages. The benefits derived by the performance of this kind of training simply cannot be overemphasized. There is however another intensive training that is used in the weight room- that which known as High-Intensity Power Training – HIPT.

The most accurate measure of aerobic conditioning is the increase of oxygen consumption. There are three weightlifting exercises that boosts the increase of oxygen - Squats, Deadlifts and Overhead Presses.

Include these three exercises for not only strength and muscle growth but for aerobic fitness, an increase of testosterone and an increase of growth hormones as well.

MUSCLE GROUP	EXERCISE	SETS	REPS	REST
BACK	BENT OVER BARBELL ROWS	4	10-12	1-2 MIN
	ONE ARM D/B ROWS	3-4	8-12	1-2 MIN
	BENTOVER TWO ARM D/B ROW	4	8-10	1-2 MIN
	INVERTED ROW	3	8-10	1-2 MIN
	T-BAR ROW	4	10	1-2 MIN
	GOOD MORNINGS	3	8-10	1-2 MIN
	DEADLIFTS	4	< 10	2-3 MIN
	BACK EXTENSIONS	3	12-15	1-2 MIN

MUSCLE GROUP	EXERCISE	SETS	REPS	REST
ABDOMINALS	PLANKS	3	1 MIN+	1-2 MIN
	SIDE PLANKS	4	15 SEC+	1-2 MIN
	CRUNCH	3	F	1-2 MIN
	REVERSE CRUNCH	3	F	1-2 MIN
	HANGING KNEE RAISE WITH TWIST	5	F	1-2 MIN
	HANGING LEG RAISE	5	F	1-2 MIN
	ARMS EXTENDED CRUNCH	10	F	1-2 MIN
	D/B SIDE BEND	2	12-15	1-2 MIN
	LEG RAISES-FLUTTER KICKS	3	<15	1 MIN

APPENDIX B

The negative side effects of Anabolic Steroids are well known to those who are serious about their health, wellness and strength. There are however certain foods that contain natural steroids that are found to boost testosterone and growth hormones. These foods contain Androgens (a male sex hormone) and other nutrients beneficial for muscle and strength:

1. Grass-fed Beef
2. Herring
3. Smoked Fish
4. Oysters
5. Celery
6. Spinach
7. Quinoa
8. Eggs
9. Fava Beans
10. Avocados
11. Extra-Virgin Olive Oil
12. Wild Oats
13. Nuts
14. Onions
15. Truffles

16. Bananas

17. Figs

18. Asparagus

19. Pine Pollen

20. Any foods high in Vitamin C, A, D, Zinc and Magnesium

Index

1. **ATP** – Short for Adenosine Triphosphate. This is found in the muscle, organic in nature and when broken down yield's energy for muscle contraction.

   CP – Short for Creatine Phosphate. This is stored in the cells and can be used to resynthesize ATP.

   Together the ATP/CP pathway is used in actions where explosive and ballistic strength and maximal effort are required. Examples of this would be powerlifting and weightlifting.

2. In addition to possibly reversing the effects of chronic conditions such as obesity and Type 2 Diabetes - both known risk factors for cancer, fasting assists in the fight against cancer by lowering insulin resistance and levels of inflammation. Source: Medical News Today

3. Source: International Sports Sciences Association

4. A 6-ounce Filet Mignon would provide 30 grams of Protein and 490 Calories.

3 oz. Wild Atlantic Salmon - 21 g. Protein, 153 calories

3 oz. Boneless, skinless Chicken Breast – 25 g. Protein, 110 calories

5. BCAAs, particularly L-Leucine help increase work capacity by stimulating production of insulin which is the hormone that opens muscle cells to Glucose. Source: ISSA

6. Our young guest, who for the life of me sounded like Michael Jackson, did not last long at the Camp. A few weeks after his arrival he was found with a cell phone. Thrown in the SHU-the Special Housing Unit (otherwise known as solitary) for a few months after which he was then transferred to a Low Facility.

7. James 1:2-3

8. "Was Mich Nicht Umbringt, Macht Mich Starker" – "That which does not kill me, makes me stronger" - Friedrich Nietzsche

9. 10,000 – 12,000 people are added to this list *every day*! The FBI's Criminal Database lists nearly 80 million Americans as criminals!! These are astounding figures. Statistics provided by the Wall Street Journal, August 18th, 2014

10. Baseball's Ty Cobb holds the highest batting average of .367 – in other words he was successful 37% of the time. Babe Ruth 34% and Michael Jordan's free throw success rate was an

amazing 83 ½ %. The conviction rate for the U.S. Department of Justice is an astounding 99.8%! Source: Info Hub

11. Written in, or around 51 AD, this scripture is found in 1 Thessalonians Chapter 5 verse 17 imploring God's people to "Pray without Ceasing".

12. Vipassana Meditation. For a complete understanding of, and guidance for performing this style of meditation I encourage you to read "Vipassana Meditation as taught by S. N. Gonka" by William Hart

13. By the autumn of 2011 when I entered prison, the federal incarceration rate had grown to over 213,000.

14. Furloughs also include being allowed to spend a certain number of hours with your family off of and away from the prison facility. Special occasions such as funerals or visiting terminally ill family members are the most common reasons Furloughs are granted. Again, white-collar inmates were routinely denied even these valid reasons.

15. I advise, *strongly advise,* against doing bench dips (traditionally performed with arms behind the back) as it requires too much internal shoulder rotation and can pinch the Rotator Cuff. Keeping the arms parallel to the body is a better way to perform dips.

16. If you decide to hire a personal trainer always insist that they are Certified. A Certified Fitness Trainer has the knowledge, training and credentials to help train and guide a client safely.

17. The International Sports Sciences Association (ISSA) recommends an increase in weight of 2% - 5% for advanced lifters and 5% - 10% for new and intermediate trainees. I received my Certification from ISSA.

18. The case against General Michael Flynn (USA v Michael T. Flynn 12/1/17 USDC District of Columbia) is but one well-documented example.

19. The three primary Anabolic Hormones in the body are Testosterone, Growth hormone and Insulin. Unfortunately, when someone hears the word "Anabolic" they think of Anabolic Steroids - Dinabol, Deca Durabolin, Winstrol and Equipoise to name a few which are illegal. Anabolic means "growth" and our bodies live in a constant state of growth and destruction. Lifting weights will naturally release beneficial hormones into the body.

BAPTISING INTO BEAST MODE

1   New muscle develops during recovery time. If you hit each body part on separate days with an all-out blitz you need time to rest those specific muscle groups. If you train the same body parts twice a week allow 48-72 hours between those sessions making one workout a heavy workout – known as work sets - and the other a lighter work set. Remember - you don't grow in the weight room. You grow at home.

2   Hit every body part during your training. Chances are the one muscle group you dislike working is the one you have the toughest workout with, consequently that's the area you need to work hardest.

3   Work for yourself. Learn from others in the weight room (a Certified Fitness Trainer is much better) but accept that each of us are genetically different and what works for another may or may not work for you. This is called "The Principal of Individual Differences" Actually there are what's called "The Seven Granddaddy Laws" of which this principal is one. To compete with a specific weight or particular move with someone else could lead to injury if you're not ready for

such a move or weight which could set you back in your training.

4 Weightlifting is a coordinated set of moves which, when done correctly, causes microscopic tears in the muscle fibers. This causes, simply put, the muscle to 'scab over' thereby increasing muscle hypertrophy - the increase in the size of the cells that make it up. Proper nutrition, plentiful hydration and abundant rest can help a person create a physique of tremendous strength and power. If possible, train each body part strenuously once a week.

5 If you want to get big you *must* squat. Legs are the biggest and heaviest muscles on the body and the most prone to respond to weight training. As the largest group of muscles, growth hormones are released as well as causing positive metabolic effects due to those large masses of muscle which burn calories even while at rest.

6 The positive effect of Cardio training could never be overstated however caution should be used in that overtraining can easily occur. Cardio work creates a lean look that most weightlifters want in order to compliment a muscular physique but the huge calorie deficit - upwards a 300 calories per workout - depletes vital muscle building components such as carbohydrates. For optimal fat-burning

and cardiovascular health, four 15 minutes sessions of High Intensity Interval Training per week - done on an empty stomach as described earlier in the book - along with a well-thought-out diet will also shed pounds quickly. For weight maintenance HIIT sessions can be limited to 3 times per week while still eating sensibly.

7   Using wrist straps offers significant advantages on pulling exercises. Using wrist straps on lifts such as 1-arm Rows, bent over rows, pull-ups and Deadlifts will give you an extra rep or two as well as allowing you to increase weight that your grip alone may not be able to hold. The muscles of the back will always benefit with the ability to add – while maintaining proper form and correct technique – weight to a pull or the ability to increase reps.

8   Abdominal and core work should not be done as the first exercise of the weight training session. Intra-abdominal pressure is that which supports the spine from collapsing forward during exercise. Lifts such as Squats, Bent-over rows and Deadlifts are dependent on a strong core and performing strenuous ab training and/or core-specific work immediately prior to a training session will fatigue and impede this critical function.

There are four main muscles that make up the abdominals - the Rectus Abdominis - those muscles in front known as the six pack. The Internal and External oblique - those muscles on the side. External near the surface and the internal located behind them. The fourth known as the Transverse Abdominis which are roughly located behind the Rectus abdominis.

Working all of these muscles will not only greatly strengthen your core and allow you to look fit but will protect your spine during strenuous exercise. If your schedule allows, you could consider doing ab work at least 5 hours before your weight training session or you could incorporate them at the end of your workout.

9   Rest and Recovery are as important as exercising. As I've stated previously - *muscles don't grow in the gym - they grow at home*. It would benefit your muscles to take a pre-planned break every 6th week and 12th week. Week 6 would have you drop your weight by half. If you're squatting 225 lbs you would lower it to 115 lbs. If your bench press is 275 lbs you reduce the weight to 135 lbs for that week and so on.

Every 12th week take the entire week off. Not only will your muscle joints and ligaments benefit from the rest, but you will be challenging yourself again as well!

The first week back would be a good time to change up your routine a bit. For example, if the previous quarter saw you doing Preacher curls you could switch to Concentration curls. If you were performing bench presses with a barbell you could now use dumbbells for the next 12 weeks.

Always challenge your muscle groups with different moves for optimal growth.

10   Consider using wrist wraps during your pushing or pulling workouts. Not to be confused with wrist *straps* which assist in gripping, wrist wraps offer a degree of stability to the wrist.

There are 8 bones in the human wrist and given the relatively small size of these bones, it's advisable to not only use wrist wraps while performing wrist curls and reverse wrist curls but to also use your opposite hand to support the wrist in use. I suggest performing these curls with dumbbells so as to allow a natural range of movement of the wrist while firmly gripping the wrist in motion with the other hand for added support.

11   Form and technique. These two words are spoken with respect by accomplished lifters due to the importance of them. Performing reps cleanly and with a proper range of motion will not only allow you to progress faster but prevents injury. Sometimes serious injury.

Too many people determine that we need to get jacked as quickly as possible which can lead to bad form during work sets. For example, instead of squatting to parallel (I personally caution you going below parallel) some may squat high, which indicates the weight being used is too heavy. A trainer can help identify the proper form, but most people can observe this on their own.

Another common mistake is performing high bench presses. Proper technique calls for the bar to touch the chest slightly before raising it back up. Be careful to not bounce the bar off the chest as well, which can assist in propelling a bit-too-heavy bar. This can cause serious injury to the ribs and sternum by cracking these bones or in more severe cases crush the chest.

Leave your ego at the gym door! Lift with weights that allow you to perform reps without breaking form.

12   A habit that some lifters have developed is to look upward while performing certain exercises - squats, shoulder shrugs and bent-over rows comes to mind. The cervical spine has a natural arch and interfering with that arch-especially with significant weight on your spine puts tremendous pressure on the spinal discs and can cause injury. Focus your eyes forward - meaning keep your head in a neutral position - about 45 degrees to the floor. Put another way direct your eyes just as a neutral spine would direct you. When you are lifting a bar from the floor – deadlifts for instance, but really any heavy object, use you legs to lift of course but do not look down as you do! This could cause the back to bow which in turn could lead to serious injury. Keep the head in a neutral position.

13   Take at least one day per week for rest and recovery. This means just enjoy the day - no lifting, no cardio. If you are

open to it, use this day as a cheat day. Observing what and when you eat during the other 6 days will usually offset the additional calories you take in on a cheat day. Going full out 7 days will take a toll on your body and could result in overtraining.

Weightlifting is considered an *anaerobic* exercise meaning that it is an intense short-term activity and derives its energy from stored internal compounds without the use of oxygen from the blood. Cardio training is an *aerobic* activity which requires oxygen in order to perform the exercise - running, cycling, rowing etc. - for more than a few minutes. Anaerobic athletes would experience sympathetic overtraining symptoms, whereas aerobic athletes are more susceptible to parasympathetic overtraining.

Sympathetic overtraining can lead to a lots of serious problems - increased blood pressure, increased resting heart rate, loss of appetite, decreased body mass, sleep disturbances, emotional instability and elevated Basal Metabolic Rate (BMR - the minimum energy required to maintain the body's life function at rest).

Parasympathetic overtraining would entail early onset of fatigue, increased resting heart rate, decreased heart rate recovery after exercise and increased resting blood pressure

Use common sense when you lift or perform cardio. Train sensibly not heedlessly.

THE 7 GRANDDADDY LAWS

For optimum effectiveness when exercising there is a group of training principals that takes into consideration the science behind that training. These principals are known as the Seven "Granddaddy" Laws.

1.   The Principal of Individual Differences

This principal acknowledges that we are all genetically different and although we may perform the same exercise movements, we will not receive the same results at the same rate or to the same extent.

2.   Overcompensation Principal

This principal acknowledges that results happen in response to stress. Muscle fibers grow as a result of exercise. Friction causes calluses to form on your hands. These are survival mechanisms encoded in our genetic make-up.

3.   Overload Principal

This principal states that in order to gain strength, muscle size and endurance we must exercise with a greater amount of weight (or resistance) than we normally would encounter. It also states that we need to continually increase the resistance so as to overcome the body's adaption to that weight. There will come a time however that the body will not be able to recuperate to keep up the increase in weight in which case the training schedule would need to change.

4.   SAID Principal

This acronym stands for **Specific Adaptation to Imposed Demands**. Simply put the SAID Principal stresses that whatever training objectives you impose on yourself must be performed in accordance with that objective. In other words, if your objective is deriving cardiovascular benefits, you must perform exercises that will burden and tax the heart. If you desire explosive strength, you must perform explosive exercises.

5.   USE / DISUSE Principal

When we train - cardio or weights - our bodies will adapt to meet the stress. When we stop training our bodies adapt to the lower stress. Unfortunately, our bodies take less time to lose muscle than it does to build muscle. Our neuromuscular system (the connection of the nervous system and muscular system) allows some training-related changes to remain over long periods.

This is what is referred to as "muscle memory" which allows a person to regain strength and size more quickly than starting from scratch.

6.   Specificity Principal

When starting a workout program most people will work foundationally. In other words, train in a general way. As a person continues to exercise, they become more focused on what direction their training should take. It may be for optimized fitness, or it could be to become an athletic competitor. The neuromuscular system will adjust over time allowing gains in strength on specific exercises. For example, a person will become stronger in Straight Leg Deadlifts by doing straight leg deadlifts as opposed to performing Romanian Deadlifts.

7.   GAS Principal

GAS short for **General Adaption Syndrome.** Basically, this principal states that after high intensity training the body must observe a period of complete rest or at the least low intensity training. This allows the muscles to heal. The 7 Granddaddy Laws disclosures courtesy of ISSA

Acknowledgements............

The 19th Century author Christian Nestell Bovee once wrote "False friends are like our shadow, keeping close to us while we walk in the sunshine, but leaving us the instant we cross into the shade". Knute Rockne, the former coach of Notre Dame observed "All the world loves a winner and has no time for a loser". Powerful observations.

If you've ever had reversals, and I mean really bad mess-ups where you lose everything, then you'll probably agree with the above statements. But like most everything in life there are hidden messages if only you stop feeling sorry for yourself and pay close attention. I was allowed to find out who my sincere friends were and who *truly* loved me. Through the most challenging time of my life, this discovery was a true blessing and one I will always be grateful for..........

I wanted to take a few moments to recognize, as well as to say "thank-you" to those who helped me, guided me, and supported me through the greatest storm of my life. I love you...........

To my editor Hannah Gordon – you took the ramblings and run-ons as well as the needless and crafted a story of health, tears, and triumph into something engaging. Thank-you so very much....

To my children Guy, Geoffrey, Jennifer and Jenna...My God what I put you all through.....you were there for the good times - Division St., Rose Circle, OOB. and so much more, but you didn't abandon me in the bad. You walked through hell with me and because of me - and through iron gates, steel bars and razor wire as well - you gave me the will to go on at the lowest point of my life. You loved me unquestioningly and supported me in every way. You truly *are* my life—always have been and always will be......

To my grandchildren-Giuliana, Gabriela and Grazia. I love you beyond words... Tuo nonno ti adora, ti ama e ti adora.......

To Alex Mouzas-you lost so much but you never deserted me. When your mother passed away on that terrible Tuesday in September 2011 you *still* boarded a plane and traveled 500 miles to speak to the court on my behalf at my sentencing the next day. Thank-you for the many articles, documents and unending favors you unhesitatingly did for me while I was inside. Thank-you *pio stenos filos* for trusting me and for always having my back. I cherish our friendship and I am honored that you are in my life…….

To Jan Hamilton and Peter BonSey - Words could never convey the love I have for you both. You NEVER gave up on me. You were there through it all and you continued to show me love and your absolute undying belief in me. You traveled for hours to see me so many times, you let me cry to you when my heart was torn apart, you got me to laugh again, you let me dream about a someday future and you never allowed me to get down on myself . You-YOU-taught me what friendship is: It's love wrapped in a noun that can never truly convey the depth nor the meaning. I love you guys always…….

When I was struggling with my eyesight in the bowels of hell Dave Christian was there. Dave - you supported me in every way as we navigated the greatest trials of our lives……thank-you my friend for showing the compassion and love that Jesus spoke of.

To Walt Olszowy - you were there and never stopped showing your support and friendship. A better friend would be hard to find. You never abandoned me and you believed in me….Thank-you my treasured friend.

Diane Shaw - you nursed me back to life emotionally and, I'm sure, didn't know it. You never knew how much I appreciated you. You greeted me with a smile in your voice every time I called. To hear that voice brightened an otherwise dreary and sad existence. Your emails uplifted me, your cards cheered me, and you helped me regain my sense of worth again…..You helped me when I could not have been lower. You will forever be in my heart. My love is with you always.

To Brenda Fire-Flataeu - I cherish you my cousin. You never forgot me. You never turned away from me. Your cards, your concern and your love never failed to fill my heart with gratitude and affection. Grazia il mio bellisima cugina. Ti amo cosi tanto…..

To Pastor Mark Gregori - My brother in Christ. Each and every time we spoke, I felt inspired, encouraged and uplifted. "For I was hungry and you gave me food; I was thirsty and you gave me drink; I was a stranger and you took me in; I was naked and you clothed me; I was sick and you visited me; I was in prison and you came to me." When we met so many years ago, I knew you were a good and decent man. A righteous man of God. You spoke up for me. You promoted me. You strengthened me. For you to travel over 3 hours to surprise me when I walked out of those prison doors, knowing that our time together would last just a few minutes - I am blessed, truly blessed, to have your friendship and love…..Thank-you my brother.

To Pastor Tim English - Each time we spoke you had a smile in your voice. You gave me your love and your friendship without judgement and without reserve. Knowing who truly loves you, believes in you and cares for you is a rare insight into a man's life and you showed and extended those gifts to me. God bless you my brother – and thank-you.

To my cousin Steve Gane – thank-you for the love and encouragement you gave me during my dark night of the soul. Your goodness and kindness have always - and will forever be - so appreciated.

Don and Laura Murley – my film editor, my brother in Christ….you are both so loved. Thank-you for being part of my life.

To those in the yard that I left behind. I promised I would not stop fighting for you. For us. *And I meant it.* Although we didn't always see eye to eye (even despite going nose to nose at times!) I am and always will be grateful for you all.

And finally, to my Lord and Savior Jesus Christ. I *always* felt Your presence. Through eyes that were filled with tears and a heart that was completely shattered and broken, you gave me the "strength that surpasses all understanding" to look to tomorrow. Without imparting that unsurpassed strength to me every moment of my confinement I could *never* have survived those sad, aching years and that torturous path………..

Guy is an example of what never giving up looks like. His commitment now is to take years off of someone's learning curve - be it a CEO, Entrepreneur, Sales Executive or Student – by imparting wisdom not borne by research but by experience. Living a complete life, he is truly the guy who has 'been there, done that'. For more information please visit him at www.ganewisdom.com

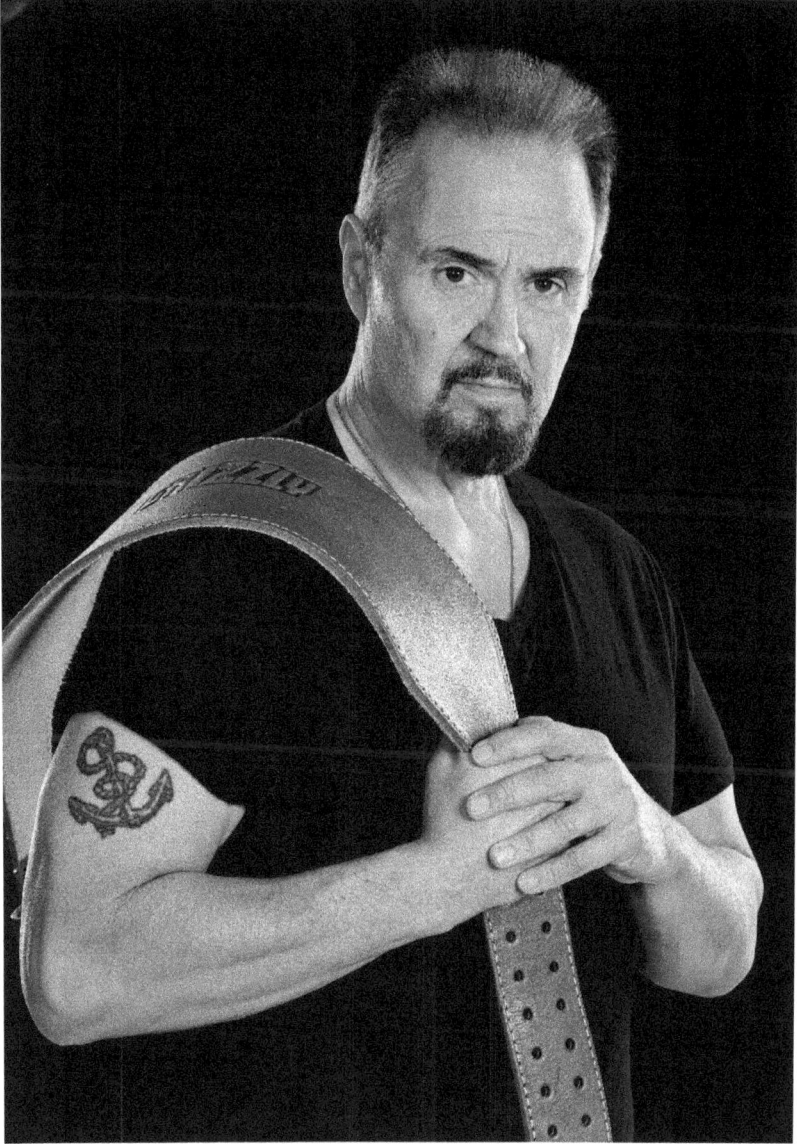

October 2021

www.ingramcontent.com/pod-product-compliance
Lightning Source LLC
Chambersburg PA
CBHW072124020426
42334CB00018B/1701